Understanding the Pancha Mahabhutas

Copyright © Yoga Satsanga Ashram UK 2021

Written by
Yogachariya Jnandev Giri

Editor & Illustrator
Yogacharini Deepika Saini

ISBN 978-1-914485-00-8

First Published June 2021

Designed, Printed & Published by Design Marque

Printed in Great Britain by www.designmarque.co.uk

Material within this book, including text and images, is protected by copyright. It may not be copied, reproduced, republished, downloaded, posted, broadcast or transmitted in any way except for your own personal, non-commercial use. Prior written consent of the copyright holder must be obtained for any other use of material. Copyright in all materials and/or works comprising or contained within this book remains with Author and other copyright owner(s) as specified. No part of this book may be distributed or copied for any commercial purpose.

With Gratitude

This book on Pancha Mahabhutas is for all the sincere Yoga, Health and Spiritual Seekers – may we all live in harmony with our truest nature.
I would like to offer my gratitude and special thanks to my dearest Guru Ammaji Meenakshi Devi Bhavanani, Swamiji and Dr Ananda Balayogi Bhavanani, along with many other true masters of yoga and Vedic culture, who have blessed me with these teachings and supported my spiritual journey.

I would like to offer my special thanks and gratitude to my Dharma Patni, Yogacharini Deepika Saini, and our three divine boys, Siddha, Mahadev and Krishna, for all their love and support as well as motivation in my life. I am also grateful for all the hard work Deepika puts into the artwork, editing, discussions and advice on various topics to bring this work to fruition.

I am very grateful to the Selfless Service (Niskama Seva) of Dharmananda for proofreading this book, and Sarah Ray (Design Marque, Pembrokeshire) for the truly amazing design work as always. Finally, I also offer my thanks to all my Yoga Family and the local Welsh community, all of whom have supported both Yoga Satsanga Ashram and me on the yoga path of teaching, writing and living a yogic life.

May we grow and evolve together!
May we all live in harmony with and within!
May we all live our full potential!
May we all attain peace and bliss!
Hari Om Tat Sat !

Yogacharya Jnandev Giri (Surender K. Saini)

Panchamahabhuta
Content List

1	Some Thoughts on Pancha Mahabhutas By Dr Ananda Balayogi Bhavanani	07
2	Pancha Bhuta: The five elements, health, and mind By Yogacharini Anandi, Cyprus.	10
3	Pancha-Maha-Bhutas – Five Major Elements Of Life	14
4	The Tattvas or Realities	16
5	The Moola-Prakriti (Basic Primordial Element)	19
6	The Pancha-Mahabhutas and their manifestation:	20
7	Dhatus and Mahabhutas	23
8	Lakshana of Mahabhutas:- Special Characteristics of the Five Elements	25
9	Mahabhuta Balancing Mudras	26
10	Pancha Mahabhuta Suddhi	34
11	Chakra Meditation for Pancha-Mahabhuta Suddhi	41
12	Pancha-Mahabhutas in Summary	48
13	Key Mantras for Pancha Mahabhutas	53
14	Asanas, Kriyas and Pranayama for Pancha-Bhutas	55
15	Key Resources	80
16	References	87
15	Glossary	88

SOME THOUGHTS ON THE PANCHA MAHABUTA

By Dr Ananda Balayogi Bhavanani

All systems of Indian philosophy (Shat Darshana etc) and healing (Ayurveda, Siddha etc) give importance to the Pancha Maha Bhuta, the five major elements of the manifest world. These are Pritvi or Bhumi (earth), Apas or Jala (water), Tejas or Agni (fire), Vayu (air), and Akasha (ether or space).

This is slightly different from the European system that focuses primarily on the first four elements neglecting Akasha that is the most subtle. The Maha Bhutas are considered the grossest manifestation in our journey from Purusha and Prakriti which is the foundation of the gross existence on this worldly plane. They are also the starting point for our return journey back home-sweet-home to the ultimate oneness of OM.

I have been contemplating the Pancha Maha Bhutas recently and have realised that these universal elements have both positive and negative connotations!

Prithvi refers to the cohesive aspects of solid material that is tightly bound together. This is the firm foundation upon which we can begin our journey. It implies a positive sense of stability but also can imply a negative stubborn refusal to change! It can often be the hard rock that prevents our growth. It can also be the worst of dirt that blemishes us and makes us impure. When people throw dirt on us, it is up to us to make it manure and utilize it to further our growth. If we don't do this, then we will be bogged down resulting in a sooner than later permanent visit to the cemetery.

Apas refers to a diplomatic ability of adaptation to the environment in a fluid manner. It is a nice 'liquid' quality and enables one to often live a comparatively "stress free" life. Water when thrown on us can either clean us or put out the fire of aspiration. Some people water the garden but most tend to try and put out the flame of creativity. Water may induce a sense of 'wishy-washy-ness' that prevents one from doing what must be done as part of one's Dharmic responsibilities. When the water finds its rightful balance it is lovely, but if not, it can create a tsunami in our growth!

Tejas can be the fire of aspiration, creativity and motivation. Yet, if one is not careful it is very easy to get burnt. There are so many who have a "fire in their belly". This thermal state can be a double-edged sword as it can motivate some to do their best but it can also create indigestion in many, resulting in 'burn out'. Fire can be the light of wisdom when it is a steady flame but it can also destroy everything if it is an unstable inferno.

Vayu may be the gentle breeze that relaxes us and reinvigorates us. It can be the inner ability to move with the flow of energy. Yet, if one is not conscious it can be the whirlwind or tornado that crates havoc everywhere. When the internal wind-like energy (Vata or Pawan) is balanced the nervous energies flow in a balanced manner and if not, great instability of the whole nervous system can destroy our health. Too much gas in the system is bad and too much of it in the ego leads to real 'bloated heads' that are none too pleasant. 'Airy fairy' types with no connection to reality abound in the world today and most need a bit of deflating by ego-dectomies. That was Pujya Swamiji's specialty, especially the ones he did without anesthesia!
Akasha is the grand space that enables us to grow in all directions and dimensions. It is the most subtle of the elements and gives us the maximum freedom. With maximum freedom comes the highest responsibility. So many of us tend to misuse freedom and think that

we are free to do the wrong things! A tendency to be scattered and lose focus on the goal is another negative aspect of this element when it is not used in a conscious and aware manner. Instead of expanding our consciousness, we may end up totally scattered and stretched out beyond our breaking point thus breaking ourselves ultimately. Giving space to people is good if they are responsible but others may need to be guided in other ways.

The final analysis of this whole concept makes us realise that the difference between the positive and negative aspects of the elements rests ultimately in our hands. If we are conscious and aware, we can maximize the positives resulting in our growth. If we choose not to do so, then the negatives will result in our destruction. The choice is ours!!

Yogacharya Dr. Ananda Balayogi Bhavanani

MBBS, ADY, DPC, DSM, PGDFH, PGDY, FIAY, MD (Alt.Med), C-IAYT, DSc (Yoga)

Yogacharya Dr. Ananda Balayogi Bhavanani is Director of the Centre for Yoga Therapy Education and Research (CYTER), and Professor of Yoga Therapy at the Sri Balaji Vidyapeeth, Pondicherry (www.sbvu.ac.in).

He is also Chairman of the International Centre for Yoga Education and Research at Ananda Ashram, Pondicherry, India (www.icyer.com) and Yoganjali Natyalayam, the premier institute of Yoga and Carnatic Music and Bharatanatyam in Pondicherry (www.rishiculture.in). He is son and successor of the internationally acclaimed Yoga team of Yogamaharishi Dr. Swami Gitananda Giri Guru Maharaj and Yogacharini Kalaimamani Ammaji, Smt Meenakshi Devi Bhavanani.

PANCHA BHUTA
The five elements, health, and mind

Human existence is made of the five elements (earth, water, fire, air, ether) not only on the material level, but also on the emotional and mental.
People think, feel, move lightly like air, intensely like fire, flow like water, are stable and earthy or hover like ether.
A balanced person "contains" all five elements almost equally.

What does this mean?

A balanced person will use the right element at the right time to face any challenge in life. Sometimes we need to be steady and strong like the earth, other times flexible and fast like the wind, other times intense and precise like the fire…!
It sounds like a bed-time-story but in fact the elements can very well become our tools for a better life!

After all, the body needs all five elements to be healthy
Element of earth for strong bones and muscles
Water element for transporting components.
Fire element for proper digestion
Air element for any movement inside and outside the body
Ether element for vitality

What can we do to sustain all the elements within us?

The proportion of the elements in us depends on the following:

1. Personal temperament (prakriti) - each person has their own character imprinted in their genes.
2. Environment, habits, personal relationships - The way we live

and with whom, also creates our temperament.
3. Breathing - the rhythm and quality of breathing is directly related to the heart and circulation, and in the long run, affects our temperament.
4. Nutrition – as we are made of the five elements, we are sustained by food which is also made by the five elements. Each food has different element ratio.

It is almost impossible to change our personal temperament only with our will, and many times it is not possible to change our environment and relationships. Therefore, what remains to achieve the balance of the elements, is to work with our breathing and nutrition.

Breathing:
Deep, slow, rhythmic breathing stabilizes the heart rhythm and balances the elements within us.
To take a deep breath, we must use all three parts of the lungs (abdominal-chest-high chest) to inhale and try to empty the lungs well on the exhale.
In order for breathing to be slow and rhythmic, it must acquire a constant rhythm. This is done only with daily practice. In our tradition of yoga, we use a specific breath ratio called Savitri Pranayama.
Savitri pranayama is also called "the balance breath" because it bring the perfect balance.
Use complete breathing (mahat yoga pranayama) to inhale for 6 seconds
Keep the breath in for 3 seconds.
Exhale for 6 seconds.
Keep the breath out for 3 seconds.
This is one round.
Practice 27 rounds and enjoy the perfect balance Savitri brings.

Diet:
The food we eat contains the five elements in proportions, so the right choice of food (which will give us more of the elements we lack and less of the elements we have) can affect our temperament. Foods contain, and create during digestion, different proportions of elements and can help us calm a strong temperament, stabilize "airy" behaviours, or "lighten up" "heavy" situations.

People who are lazy, sluggish, indecisive with lung problems or obesity problems, have an excess of earth and water elements (kapha dosha) and have to take ether, air and fire foods to compensate. These foods are; hot peppers, onions, green vegetables, sour fruits, lightly cooked foods without much oil, raw salads. If the food you eat is inappropriate for your temperament, add hot pepper to reduce the reaction.

People who are hyperactive, unstable, unconcentrated, with problems in the intestines or the nervous system, have an excess of air and ether elements (vata dosha) and have to take fire, water and earth food to compensate. These foods are; Tomato, lemon, celery, carrot, sweet potato, olives (not bitter), sweet fruit, cooked food with oil, rice, black pepper, egg, cheese. If the food you eat is inappropriate for your temperament, add lemon to reduce the reaction.

Intense, angry people, with stomach or skin problems, have an excessive element of fire and water and must take earth, air, and ether food to compensate. These foods are; coriander, parsley, green vegetables, sweet fruits, potatoes, zucchini, rice, wheat and wheat products, tofu, raw salads. If the food you eat is unsuitable for your temperament, add fresh coriander to reduce the reaction.

The five elements are contained within us, but also in the food we eat, and since "we are what we eat, what we think and what we feel", let us try to work with the method of the "opposite attitude" – (pratipaksha bhavana) that is, to give the opposite of this which excels, to balance.

Yogacharini Anandhi – Korina Kontaxaki
Holistic Spiritual Training
Activated Vegan Food seminars

Pancha-Maha-Bhutas – Five Major Elements of Life

Any of the aspects of Yoga we study, we need to know the basic principles along with the application, adaptation and practicability to succeed in our endeavours. In this lesson we are aiming to study the concepts and principles of Pancha-Mahabhutas and the simple yoga practices to enhance our healing process and well-being.

Samkhya Yoga, Hindu Darshana and Ayurveda details the theory and practices around Pancha Mahabhutas. Whole universe is within each living being and each living being is in whole universe according to Vedic teachings. Knowing this Oneness or Union is the pathway to absolute liberation. Our body is known to be composed of a modification of the Pancha-Mahabhutas. Hence the understanding of Pancha-Mahabhutas may carry a subtle understanding of our health and wellness.

Theory of Tri-Doshas, Tri-Gunas, and Rasa Sidhanta (theory of six tastes) etc were primarily based on this theory of five major elements. These five are:

1. Prathvi: - Earth or solid
2. Apa or Jala: - Liquid or water
3. Tejas or Agni: - Heat, energy or fire
4. Vayu: - Wind or air
5. Akasha: - Voidness or space

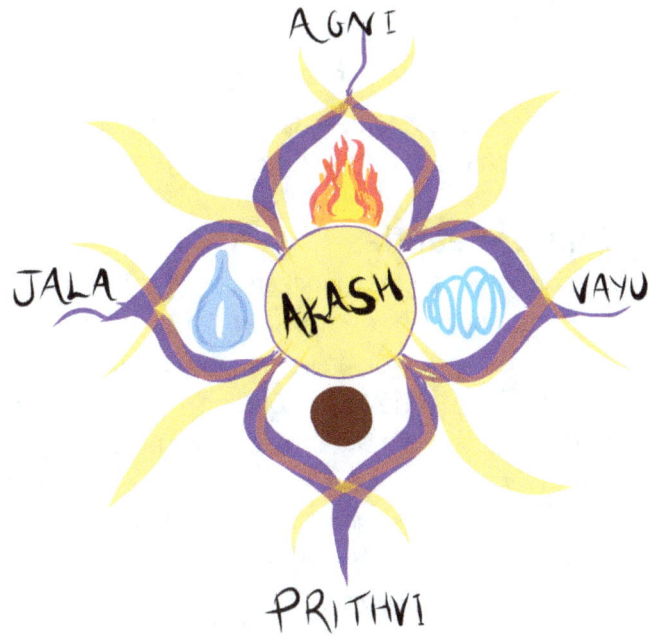

In Indian Wisdom traditions, the Vedas are considered to be the first recorded sources of this science and knowledge (Vijnana). The Vedas explain how to perform our Dharma and Karma along with religious rituals, sacrifices and ceremonies for health, evolution, prosperity and peace.

Samkhya, Yoga, Ayurveda and Vedantic teachings, which were developed much later on, explain in a scientific way the creation, evolution and process of life at a very subtle to gross level. I personally view these Vedic sciences as the mother of our modern sciences. Here it is explained that:

- every cause follows an effect and reaction in our living, dynamic universe.

- Each human being is a structural and functional model of the whole universe (Yat Pinde Tat Brahmande).

Parinama Sidhanta (theory of evolution or transformation) of cosmogenesis is the most widely accepted theory among various Vedic theories of creation.

The Tattvas or Realities

Prakriti (primordial nature) manifests everything through the processes of modification or transformation by the means of "the causes into effects, which are already hidden within them". Eg. Once the seed finds the ideal conditions to grow it becomes and transforms into the potential held within the seed (an acorn will become an Oak). In this example the cause and effect are the environment conditions for a seed to grow into a Tree. With various combinations of Tri-Gunas and various Tattvas, Prakriti manifests all the living and non-living objects.

It is known that Prakriti has no control or power over the Purusha or Soul. The Soul is eternal, independent, immutable, all-pervading and all-knowing. Life forms or species are created out of the Tattvas with the involvement of the Soul. This creation of Shristi or the universe begins due to the loss of the equilibrium of the Gunas in Prakriti.Gradually this evolutionary process manifests Tattvas.. In this concept 24 Tattvas or Realities evolve out of the Prakriti. Each of them has the predominance of one or more of the Gunas. These are:

1. Prakriti, Nature
2. Mahat, the greatest intellect-principle
3. Buddhi, discriminating, reasoning and causative intelligence
4. Ahamkara, ego or ego-principle
5. Manas, the physical mind or brain
6. The Pancha-Indiryas, five sense organs

7. The Karma-Indriyas, the five organs of action
8. The five tanmatras, subtle elements
   (sound, touch, smell, taste, sight)
9. The Pancha Mahabhutas, five great elements
   (the earth, water, air, fire and ether)

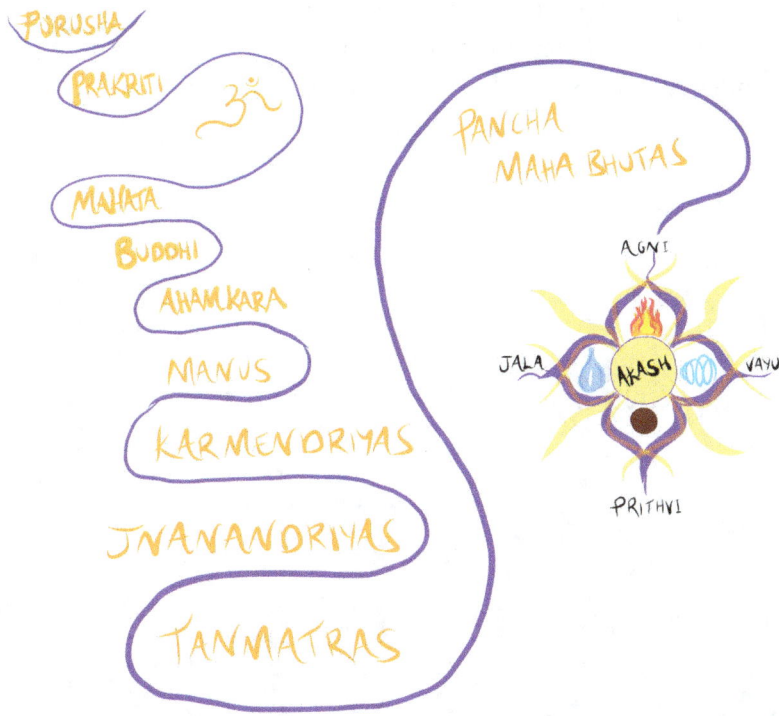

This theory draws from Sukshma or the subtle to Sthula or the gross. The evolutes of Prakriti or Tattvas, in conjunction with Purusha, create our body and life. Yogic techniques are the scientific tools to reverse this process to return back to our primordial Prakriti or attain oneness (Samadhi) in our Real Reality.

According to this Samkhya theory life evolves from the Prakriti (primordial) and Purusha (eternal consciousness). The Vaisesika theory of creation is based on atomic theory or Paramanuvada. Ayurveda has merged both of them together. These theories correlate to the modern Big Bang theory of creation. Prakriti shows a resemblance to the 'cosmic egg' idea of modern science as the sole source of the creation of the universe. It is interesting that Samkhya mentions "Hiranya-Garbha", "the golden womb of the creative Mother Nature" as the source of creation.

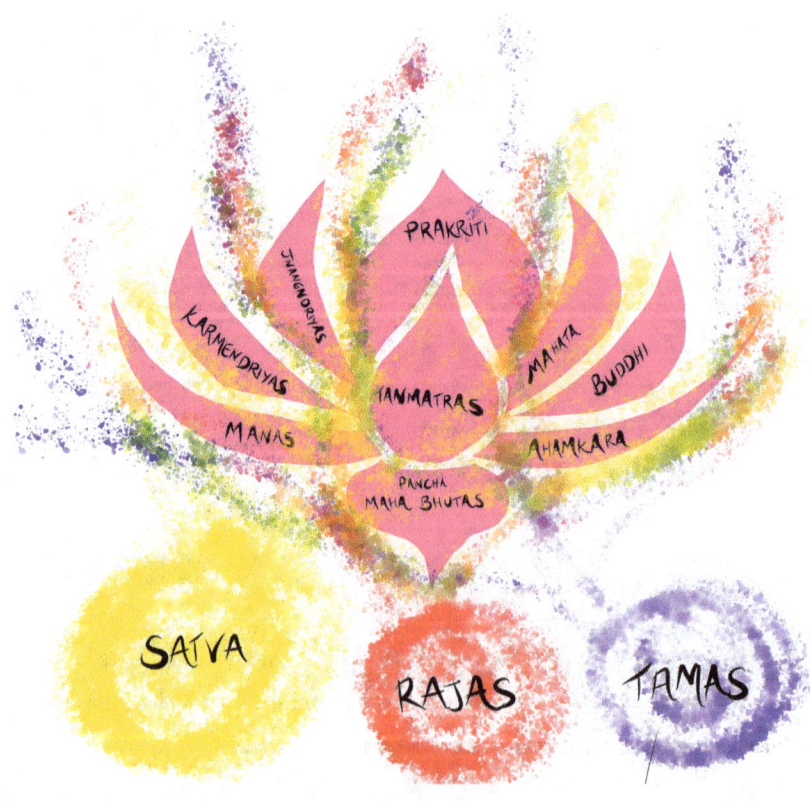

The Moola-Prakriti (Basic Primordial Element)

The inherited or inert principle of matter is the cause of all living and non-living objects by the three Gunas and Ashta Prakriti (eight primordial elements) and is the primordial unit and entity of evolution. Throughout all the Sthavara (non-living) and Jangama (living) Srishti (universe), there is a combination of Sattva (involutionary or liberating), Rajas (transforming) and Tamas (inertia or holding). These Gunas are continuously in changing proportions to sustain the dynamic and transforming process of the universe.

The combination or Samyoga of Prakriti and Purusha eternally resides in Avyakta (the unmanifest). Mula Prakriti cannot manifest life on its own. Elements cannot manifest the mind etc.

The Mahat: The Mahat or Principle Intellect Field of Chetana or consciousness becomes the first evolute which is also known as the `buddhi-tattva'. This is the intelligent principle of universal process. Think of the solar system where each of the planets and sun are moving and held effortlessly. A seed grows into a tree and recreates more seeds, takes what it needs to take from nature and still maintains the finest balance with nature. These processes are governed by the 'Mahat'.

The Ahamkara: Mahata manifests Ahamkara or the Ego or driving force of the life process. Ahamkara is divided into the Sattvika, Rajasika, and Tamasik in nature.

Ekadasa-Indriyas (eleven faculties of experience): Through Ahamkara, the manas or the mind manifest, dominated by the Tri-Gunas through which the five sense organs (Jnana-Indriyas) and five action organs (Karma-Indriyas) manifest. These sense organs are capable of bringing experience or perception of objects in conjunction with the mind.

Tanmatras (five attributes): These are five basic attributes of the sense organs, which manifest the Pancha-Mahabhutas.

The Pancha-Mahabhutas and their manifestation:

Akasha Mahabhuta: Akasha, voidness, ether or space is Vyapaka (all pervasive) and sabda-gunavisista (has special qualities of sound) and is Nitya or permanent in Nature. According to the Upanishads Atman is the original source of Akasha.

Imbalance of Akasha in general is associated with Vata Dosha. Cells are the powerful source of electromagnetic radiation and the metabolic processes in them are the constant source of free photons (light). The micro-space around the cells is not just an empty space, but the information-rich "world" in which cells exchange "data" not only through the hormones and neurotransmitters, but also through "field interaction". Hence an imbalance of the Akasha element can cause metabolic disorders and cancers as cells lose the ability to communicate in a healthy manner with other cells around them.

Vayu Mahabhuta: Vayu is the Second mahabhuta to evolve from the Sparsa Tanmantra (object of touch). Vayu also holds the qualities of Sabda Guna or sound.

Vayu is Rajo Guna dominant without which satva and tamas cannot proceed to perform their functions.

Vayu governs the movement of all things in the universe — from subatomic particles to huge rotating galaxies. Vayu is the governing principle behind the movement of nerve impulse, blood flow, muscle contraction, secretion of glands etc.

Imbalance of Vayu is associated with Vata Dosha. Vayu imbalance may lead to excessive dryness of the skin, soft tissues and joints. It can also cause an excess of cold and high sensitivity to drafts, insufficient blood flow, bloating, constipation, fatigue, insomnia, spasms, loss of emotional flexibility, a dry cough etc.

Agni Mahabhuta: The Agni is the third mahabhuta to evolve from Rupa tanmatra (Object of vision). Agni along with the vision also possess the qualities of sound and touch.

Agni is Satva & Rajo guna dominant as it derives gunas from the above Akasha and Vayu.

The main attribute of Agni is a transformation (conversion) and extracting energy from the dense matter with its subsequent involvement in the processes of growth and development. The basic qualities of Agni are heat and light.

In the human body Agni Bhuta has several forms of manifestation. In our body, Agni manifests in processes like metabolism. It is through Agni that the body is able to extract Prana (energy) from food - due to Pachaka Pitta.

According to Frank Ros, 2005, "Agni imbalance typically manifests itself as its excess, which is usually associated with fever in the body. Herewith the clinical symptoms are: increase of the body temperature, hyperacidity, skin redness, inflammation of the tissues, excessive sweating, irritability. These states are similar to the problems that arise at the excess of Pitta Dosha".

A lack of Agni is manifested in the reduction of the digestive fire, which creates problems associated with digestion of food, absorption of nutrients and excretion of toxins in the body (ama).

Lack of energy, lethargy, physical weakness, indigestion, lack of drive, depression, anxiety, fear, etc. can also be associated with Agni imbalance.

Jala-mahabhuta: The Jala is fourth in the row, originated out of Rasa Tanmatra (Object of taste). Its primary quality is taste along with sound, touch and vision as secondary qualities.

The main governing principle of Jala is the cohesion (coupling) of corpuscular particles with each other i.e. this is the physico-chemical coupling strength of electrons, atoms, molecules, forming dense matter. Another quality inherent in Jala is fluidity (the movement of delocalized electrons and other corpuscular particles), that's why it is associated with water.

Imbalance of Jala or liquid is one of the reasons for Kapha Dosha imbalance. Clinically, it can lead to hypersecretion of mucus, coughing phlegm, swelling of glands, tumour in joints, oedema in tissues, dehydration, muscular stiffness, pain, obesity etc.

Prithvi Mahabhuta: This is the fifth element to manifest with Gandha (smell) as visesha guna with all the Gunas of Preceding bhutas. Any object having mass and shape has predominance of Prithvi. Prithvi Mahabhuta is Tamo guna predominant and provides stability.

Prithvi is associated with Kapha Dosha with the manifestation of its properties of gravity and static character.

Excess of Prithvi Bhuta is manifested as colds, occlusion of blood vessels, loss of flexibility, gravity and lack of fluidity.

Shortage of Prithvi Bhuta causes decreased muscle tone, leaching of calcium from the bones, feeling of weakness.

Tridosha & Panchamahabuta: As the tridoshas are the Karya-dravyas (Products), they too are Panchabhoudhika in nature but with the predominance of one or two Mahabhuta which influences their nature and functions.

Dosha	Bhuta
Vata	Vayu +Akasha
Pitta	Agni +Jala
Kapha	Jala+Prithvi

Dhatus and Mahabhutas: Ayurveda recognizes seven physical components or systems in our body known as Dhatus. These are: rasa (plasma i.e. serum, white blood cells, lymphatic system), rakta (red blood cells), mamsa (muscle), medda (fat), asthi (bones and cartilage), majja (bone marrow, nerve tissue, connective tissue), shukra/artava (male/female reproductive organs).

According to Ashanga-samgraha, predominance of Bhutas in our body constitution is as below:

Body Constituent (Ayurveda)	Bhuta	Body Part
Rasa	Jala	plasma i.e. serum, white blood cells, lymphatic system
Rakta	Agni	red blood cells
Mamsa	Prithvi	muscle
Meda	Jala + Prithvi	fat
Asthi	Vayu	bones and cartilage
Majja	Jala	bone marrow, nerve tissue, connective tissue
Sukra	Jala	male/female reproductive organs

Lakshana of Mahabhutas:- Special Characteristics of the Five Elements are:

Bhuta	Special Characteristic
Prithvi	Kharatwa (Solidity)
Jala	Dravatwa (Liquidity)
Vayu	Chalatwa (Mobility)
Agni	Usnatwa (Hotness)
Akasha	Apratighatatwa (Unobstructiveness)

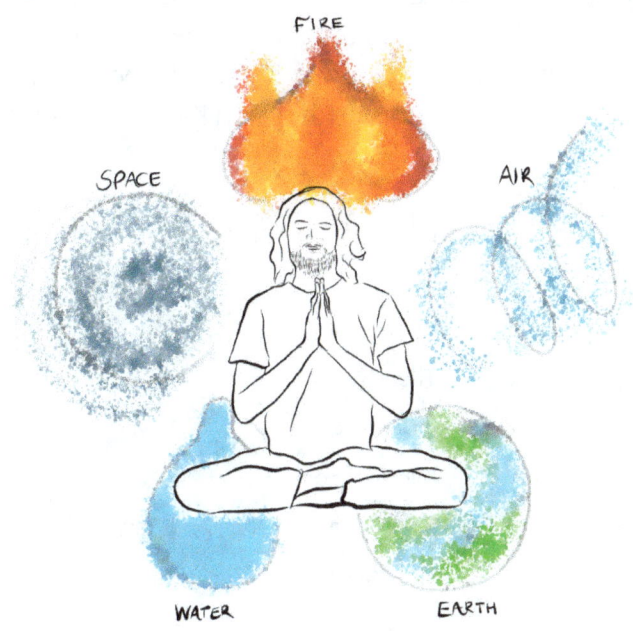

Mahabhuta Balancing Mudras

Our universe and our body both comprise of five basic elements or building elements known as Prithvi, Jala, Agni, Vayu and Akasha. Each of these elements are associated with a sense organ – the earth with the nose, water with the tongue, fire with the eye, air with the skin and space with the ear.

According to Ayurveda, many health issues are caused due to disharmony between the three doshas – Vata, Pitta and Kapha, which are also composed of five elements. Doshas determine the fundamental constitution of an individual and sustain the human body. Vata dosha is caused by an imbalance between Vayu and Akasha; Pitta dosha by Agni and Jala; and Kapha dosha by Jala and Prithvi.

Each of the fingers in our hands are also associated with the Bhutas:

Finger in Sanskrita	English	Bhuta
Angustha	Thumb	Agni
Tarjani	Index finger	Vayu
Madhyama	Middle finger	Akasha
Anamika	Ring finger	Prithvi
Kanistha	Little finger	Jala

Tips of each finger emit or release a particular pranic energy or electromagnetic energy naturally associated with a particular subtle energy current (Prana Vayu) and Bhutas according to Yoga and Ayurveda. There are more than 108 Mudras or energy seals in Yoga, dance and ceremonial acts within Yoga and Hinduism. There is an amazing set of Bhuta Mudras using our fingers to purify and balance the composition of Pancha-Mahabhutas in the body for health and wellness.

The thumb is associated with the character and is used in almost all mudras: the upper phalange signifies willpower, the lower phalange signifies logic. The ring finger is associated with the sun and represents art and beauty. The little finger is the finger of Mercury; it stands for intelligence, dexterity and consistency.

The fingertips of every living being have many nerve root endings which are energy discharge points. Science and energy readers have also shown that around every tip there is a concentration of free electrons. By touching the fingertips to each other, and to other parts of the palms, this free outward flowing energy, known as Prana, is redirected back into the specified energy channels (Nadis or Naris), back up to the particular part of body and brain. The redirected energy traveling through the nerves stimulates the various chakras.

The pressure applied to the nerves, and the neural or psycho-neural circuits formed by the mudras, help in balancing the Pancha-Maha-Bhutas. Mudras also lead to redirection of the internal energy which positively effects the changes in veins, tendons, glands and sensory organs, to bring the body back to a healthy state. Keeping specified nerves stimulated or active by means of Mudras for specified periods tones up of the nervous system.

1. Prithvi Mudra

Join the tips of the ring finger and the thumb and keep the other three fingers relaxed and straight.

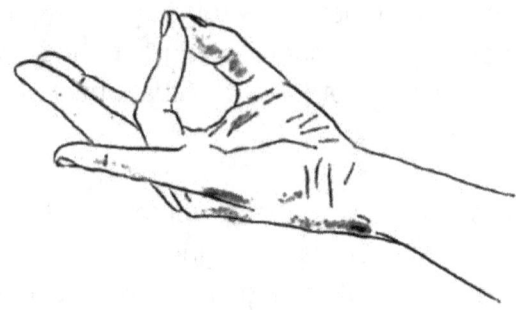

Prithvi Mudra

Benefits of Prithvi Mudra
- Good for dealing with skin diseases and rashes
- Strengthens the tissues in the body
- Helps with premature greying and hair loss
- Promotes weight gain
- Helps to overcome fatigue and nervousness
- Strengthens the bones and is therefore helpful for those affected by osteoporosis and Arthritis

2. Varuna Mudra

Gently touch the tip of the little finger and the tip of the thumb together, keeping the other three fingers relaxed and straight.

The name for this Mudra comes from the Sanskrit word Varun, which is the name of the Hindu god of water. It is also known as jal-vardhak mudra, which comes from the Sanskrit jal, meaning "water", and vardhak, meaning "enhance".

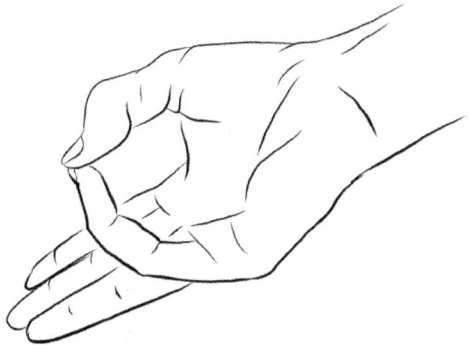

VARUNA MUDRA

Benefits of Varuna Mudra
- Relieves digestive issues like indigestion and constipation
- Helps in healing skin disorders such as eczema and psoriasis
- Provides relief to those affected by osteoarthritis
- Helps fight against Anaemia and other blood-related health issues
- Provides relief from disorders related to the bladder and kidneys
- Helps against dehydration
- Provides relief with involuntary contraction of muscles and cramps.

3. Vayu mudra
Fold your index finger and press the back of the second phalanx bone with the tip of your thumb. Apply gentle pressure so that the tip of index finger should touch the base of the thumb. Keep the other three fingers straight and relaxed.

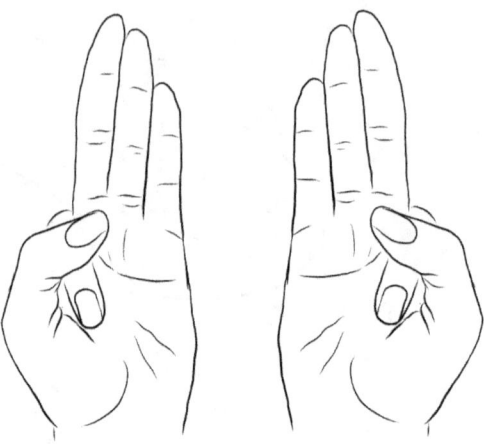

Vayu Mudra

Benefits of Vayu Mudra

- Relief from wind/gas, bloating
- Easing of constipation
- Relief from cervical spondylosis
- Brings some relief from arthritis, gout, Parkinson's disease
- Relieves chest pain
- Develops immunity against colds and coughs

4. Agni or Surya Mudra

Bend your ring finger inward and place the tip at the base of the thumb and gently press the second phalanx bone with the thumb. Keep the other three fingers straight but relaxed.

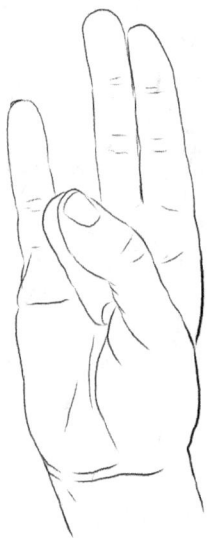

AGNI/SURIYA MUDRA

Benefits of Surya Mudra
- Reduces bad cholesterol
- Helps with weight loss by dissolving extra fat
- Enhances metabolism and energy levels
- Improves digestion
- Enhances Prana, willpower and determination
- Produces Tejas or lustre to the skin

5. Akasha Mudra
Place the tips of the middle finger against the tips of the thumbs on each hand gently, with keeping the other fingers straight and relaxed.

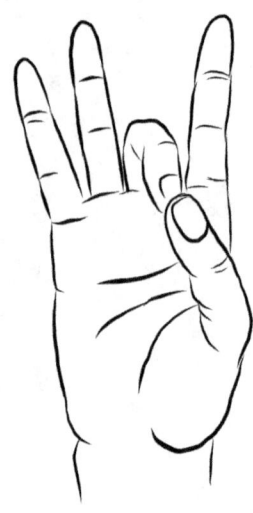

Akasha Mudra

As the element of space is all-pervading, Akasha mudra helps regulate the:
kshaya : deterioration, weakening.
vriddhi: aggravation or increase, or
prasara: expansion, of all types of doshas in the body.

Benefits of Akasha Mudra
- Connects the mundane mind to the cosmic consciousness
- Develops spiritual experiences
- Develops positive thoughts and attitudes
- Relieves negative thoughts, anger, fear, traumas, guilt and other negative emotions
- Detoxifies the body
- Eases discomfort due to overeating
- Relief from arrhythmia, chest pain and high blood pressure.

Aakash mudra activates the visuddha chakra, which governs communication, self-expression, truth and purification.

6. Prana mudra
Softly place the tip of the ring finger and the little finger against the tip of the thumb while keeping the other two fingers (index and middle) straight and relaxed.

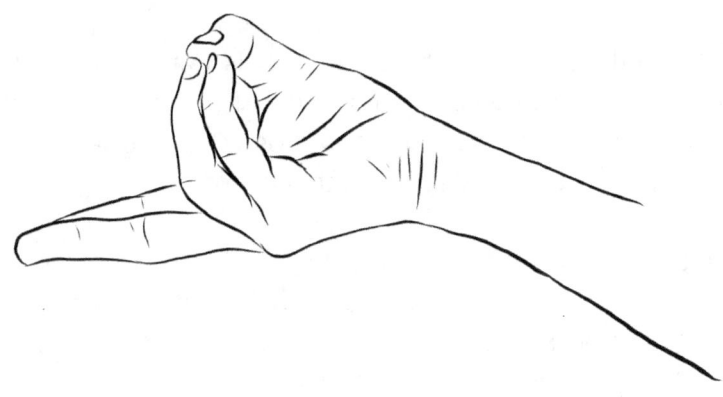

Prana Mudra

Benefits of Prana Mudra
- Enhances the immune system
- Improves the flow of vital pranic energy currents in the body
- Relieves blood pressure
- Improves vision and eyesight
- Helps encourage proper blood circulation
- Relieves mental tension, anger, restlessness, frustration
- Soothes the digestion system, relieves acidity and gastric issues

Pancha Mahabhuta Suddhi

In typical ancient Tantric and spiritual traditions, it was considered important to purify or balance the Pancha-Mahabhutas before any advanced mystical sadhana to prepare our body, Nadis, mind, and Chakras. This aims to attain the fundamental balance or nature we are born with to fulfil our Dharma and Karma in this particular life. Most of the body is composed of water, just like our Mother Earth, and the rest is comprised of earth, air, fire and Akasha or etheric voidness.

It is known that around 72% of the body is water or Jala. Twelve percent of our body composition is the earth element. Six percent of our body is Vayu or wind while four percent is Agni or fire. The remaining six percent is Akasha or etheric voidness.

Due to the imbalance of Dosha and the imbalance in our primordial qualities (Gunas), our Bhutas are also imbalanced which affects our anatomy and physiology in an adverse manner, causing physical, mental and emotional health issues. Bhuta Suddhi is a Yogic process to become free from the taint or imbalance of these five major constitutional elements in our body. Most of these days are caught up in physiological and psychological process which makes our present body, mind and Samaskaras.

Our anatomical, physiological and psychological process are governed by Gunas or qualities of our existential nature of being. If you are seeking health, balance and to access the spiritual dimensions of absolute wisdom, you need to connect with these Pancha-Mahabhutas or building-blocks of your existence.

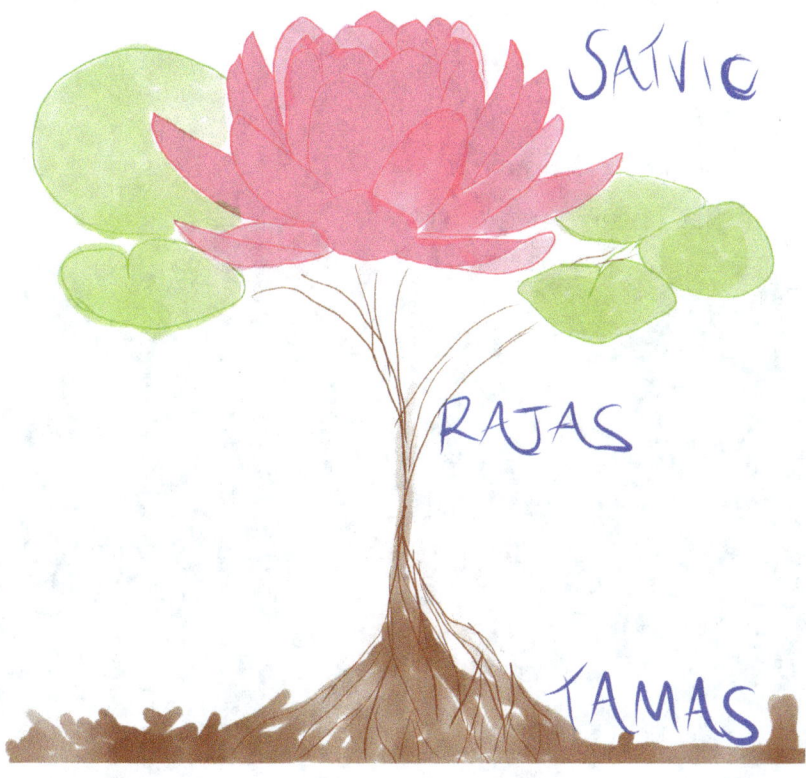

How to Cleanse the Five Elements

Jala or Water
Among all the Bhutas, Jala is the most significant as it forms the largest percentage of our body. Water holds a great amount of energy in the form of waves or prana and a sense of memory and flow. Water is actually life-producing material and holds an immense amount of potentials. So it is important to learn how we treat and consume water.

We need to not only drink pure water free from toxins, but also learn a few things such as:

How to keep water?

What is the source of water?

How long has it been stored?

Where has it been stored?

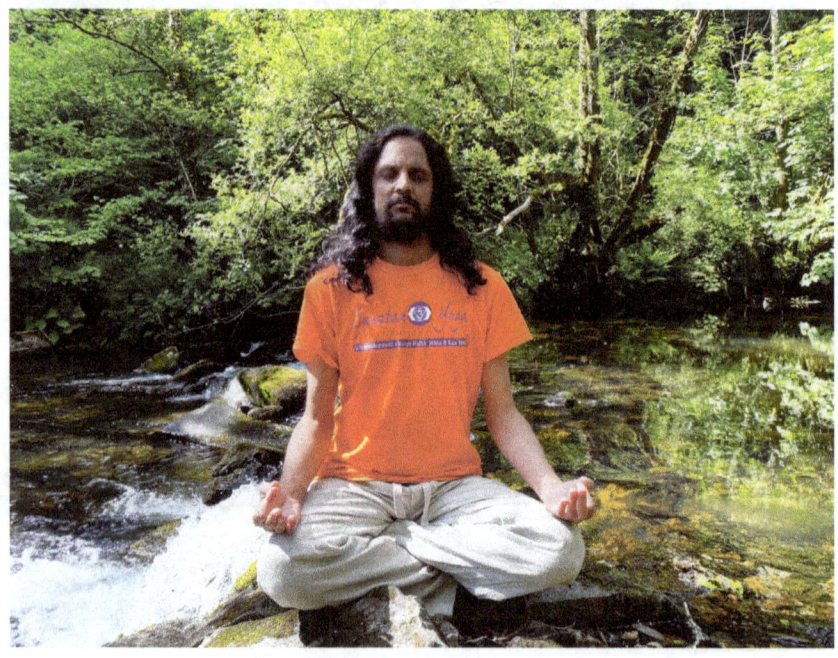

Ideally, it is best to drink fresh water from the source nearest to the place where you live. Fresh spring water or naturally flowing water is highly charged with living Prana. If you are living in a city where you rely on tap water, try to store the water overnight in a copper pot or clay pot to let it get charged up with living Prana. Avoid plastic bottled water if possible as it carries many toxic elements which causes water imbalance. Also try to create a positive thought, attitude and vibe around your drinking water, so it comes alive and develops healing properties.

Food is a great source of water. Our food should contain more than 70% water - that was one of the many reasons in Vedic times that great Rishis and Yogis promoted a vegetarian diet. Vegetables contain more than 70% water, which is perfectly aligned with the constitutional composition of our body. We should try to avoid any dry foods if possible. Many fruits contain even larger amounts of water than vegetables. Fruit fasting is highly recommended to cleanse our body and balance the Pancha-Mahabhutas.

According to Swamiji Dr Gitananda Giri, to align our constitutional body to the environment in which we are living we should try to eat the local food, take a dip in a flowing river, sea, lake or use the local fresh water for a shower or bath.

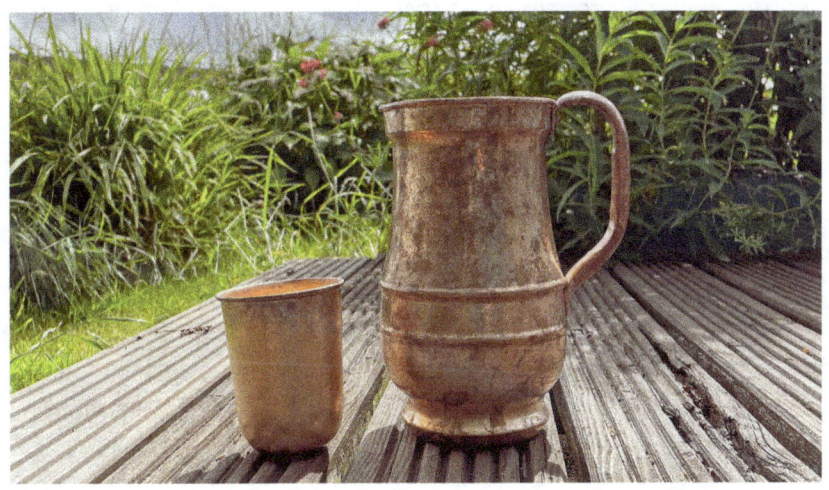

Prithvi or Earth

Prithvi includes solid material. Our Mother Earth has her own intelligence and memory. If you live in big cities and concrete blocks, it is important to find connection or touch with the living nature and qualities of earth. Take a barefoot walk in nature, or find opportunities to touch the earth with your hands and feet. Naturopathy uses mud baths to treat many health issues and to balance the earth element. Also try to interact with the plants and trees around you, seeing them as the fundamental basis of human life - a source of food, fresh air, shelter and fire.

Vayu or Air

Even though Vayu makes up a very small percentage of our physical composition, it is a dynamic element in terms of our movement, transformation and life processes. Fresh air, charged with prana in nature, will help regain the constitutional purification of the Vayu element. Vayu can also be balanced or activated by means of various Pranayama and conscious breathing.

If you are living in a big city, full of pollution and toxic air, you easily get depleted and imbalanced with regards to the Vayu element and living Prana that we receive by means of our breath. Try to go for a long walk in nature, in and around parks, in a forest, by the river or lake or sea. When the air flows along the trees or by a natural source of water, it is not only rich in oxygen but also contains an abundance of activated Prana, which helps purify all five major elements.

Try to practice some dynamic Kriyas, such as Surya Namaskar, with rhythmic breathing out in nature as many times as possible every week to enhance your physical strength, mobility, endurance and mental stability. A mountain walk or climb, a swim in the river or sea and listening to the sound of the wind are all great tools to purify our Vayu element.

Agni or Fire

Agni is another one of the Bhutas or constitutional elements in our makeup. It is worth reflecting on what kind of fire burns within us. Do you find yourself burning in anxiety, fear, worries, anger, hatred, resentment or are you full of love, compassion, care, and joy? Our Agni element is the source of our life force, mental willpower, determination and heat that we need to enact, respond with or perform in day to day life. Our health and well-being blossoms when the Agni or fire element is balanced and at its best. Hatha Yoga, Pranayama, regular exposure to sunlight along with a nutritional diet can help us to regain the Suddhi, or purity, and balance of Agni.

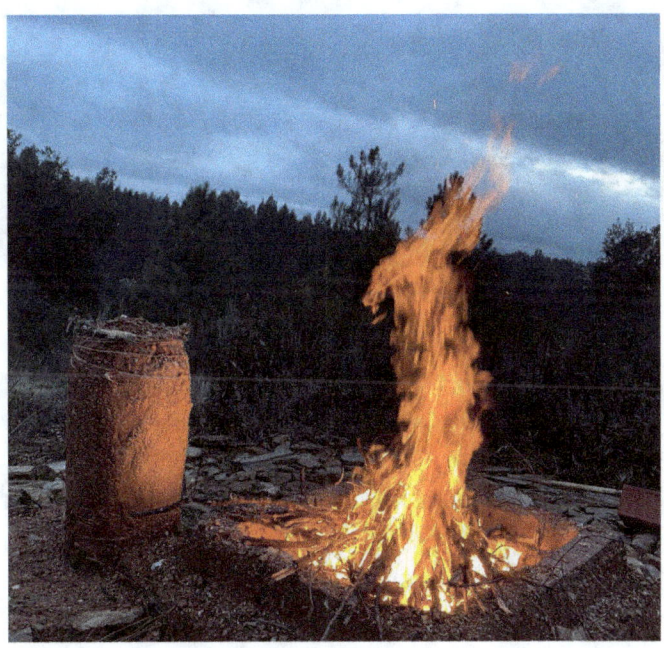

Ancient Yogis and Sadhus always kept the fire (Dhuna or Yajna – fireplace in an ashram) going to keep the fire of spiritual life active. We can also sit by a natural fire, light a candle or oil lamp around us and meditate for few minutes. This process will also help cleanse your aura and purify the Pranamaya Kosha, through which we are connected with the cosmic energy.

Akasha or Etherical Voidness

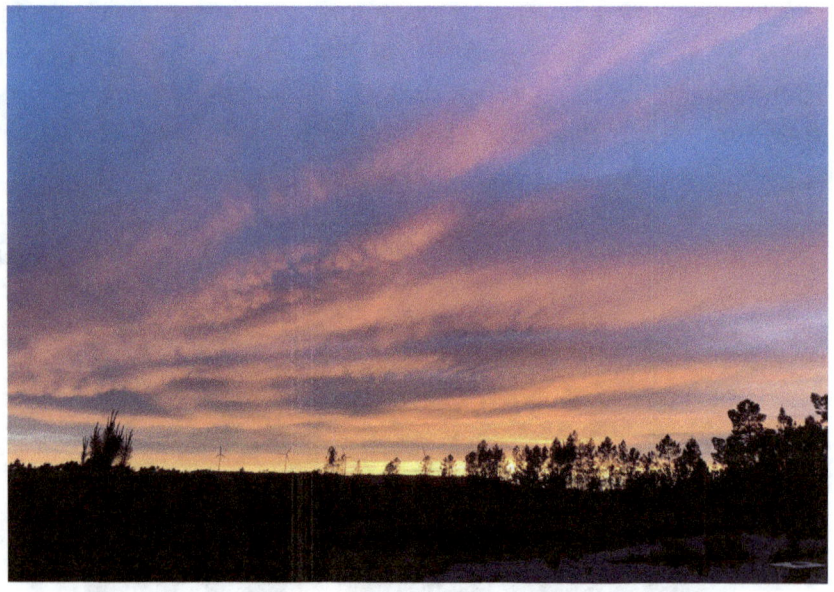

Akasha is the subtlest and ever-expanding element in our constitutional composition. Akasha holds all the cosmic wisdom known as Akashik-readings. The innermost qualities, power and nature of our life is determined by the quality of our access to the Akashik wisdom. Unlike the other four elements, Akasha is unlimited, and all-connecting. The Akasha element also gives us access to spiritual dimensions and the healing powers of life.

One of the simplest practices is to regularly witness the sky during sunrise and sunset. Naad Bindu Jnana Kriya is another powerful sadhana to enhance the access to Akasha Bhuta. Find a space somewhere in nature and listen to the sounds of wind, water, birds, leaves etc. Follow your focus from the nearest to the furthermost sound and vice versa, choosing to pay all your attention to one particular sound among all other sounds.

Chakra Meditation for Pancha-Mahabhuta Suddhi

Pancha-Mahabhutas and Chakras

Pancha-Mahabhutas and Chakras

Chakra	Bhuta	Quality
Mooladhara	Prithvi	smelling, and elimination
Swadhisthana	Jala	Tasting and procreating
Anahata	Vayu	Feelings, holding, and grasping
Manipura	Agni	Seeing, and moving
Vishuddha	Akasha	Communication
Ajna	Manas	Perception
Sahashrara	Chetana or Atman	Consciousness

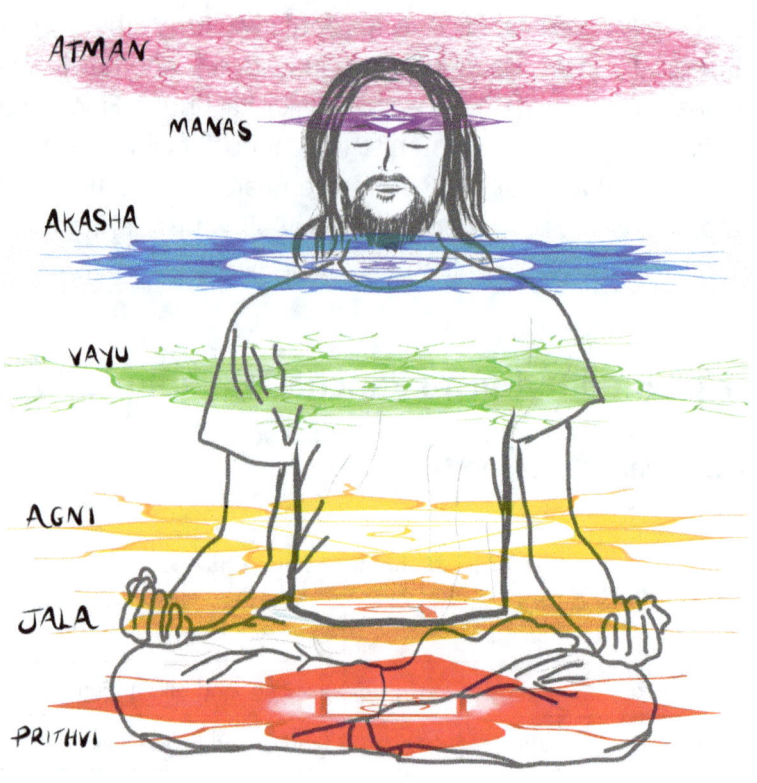

Our first five Chakras, from the Mooladhara to Vishuddha Chakra, are associated with the five major elements of creation. Each of these Chakras' primary mandala spins or resonates to access the cosmic vital force to sustain the anatomical, physiologic, psychological and spiritual life process associated with them. Chakra Meditation with colour visualisation and Bija Mantra will not just help activate these subtle energy wheels but also purify and balance our Bhutas to bring health, well-being and balance from our gross to subtlest levels of existence.

Chakra, Elements, Indriyas and Tanmatras

Chakra, Elements, Indriyas and Tanmatras

Chakra	Element	Jnanedriya	Tanmatra	Karmendriya
Sahashrara	Consciousness	Consciousness	Self-realisation	non
Ajna	Mind	Mind	Perception or cognition	non
Vishuddha	Space	Ears	hearing	Speech
Anahata	Air	Skin	Touch	Hands
Manipura	Fire	Eyes	Vision	Feet
Swadhisthana	Water	Tongue	Taste	Reproduction organs
Mooladhara	Earth	Nose	Smell	Excretory organs

Chakra, Bhuta Mandala, Colour and Bija Mantra

Chakra, Bhuta Mandala, Colour and Bija Mantra

Chakra	Bhuta Mandala and Color	Color of Bhuta Mandala	Bija Mantra
Sahashrara		Violet	OM
Ajna	Circle	Orange	ONG
Vishuddha	Oval	Magenta	HAM
Anahata	Two Intersected Triangle	Blue	YAM
Manipura	Reverse Triangle	Red	RAM
Swadhisthana	Crescent Moon	Silver	VAM
Mooladhara	Square	Yellow	LAM

Bhuta Suddhi - Chakra Meditation Process

Savitri Pranayama: Sit straight in a comfortable Asana and relax your body and mind with a few minutes of 6x3x6x3 Savitri or Solar rhythm Pranayama. (inhale 6 x hold in 3 x exhale 6 x hold out 3 by counting with the clock or your heartbeat)

Swadhisthana Chakra: Softly focus your mind across your pelvic area, gradually bringing it to the middle point, and then visualise a vibrant silver crescent moon mandala across your pelvis. Softly breathe in this mandala by chanting the Bija Mantra VAM in your mind. Repeat this for 2 to 3 minutes.

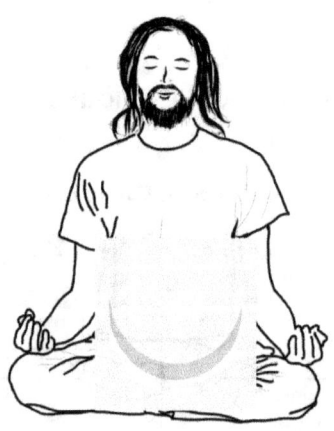

Manipura Chakra: Softly focus your mind across your stomach area/ Manipura Chakra, gradually bringing it to the middle point, and then visualise a vibrant red triangle mandala pointing downward across your abdomen with the navel in the middle. Softly breathe in this Mandala by chanting the Bija Mantra RAM in your mind. Repeat this for 2 to 3 minutes.

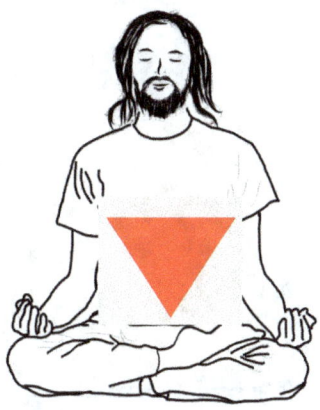

Anahata Chakra: Softly focus your mind across your thoracic area and gradually bring it to the middle point and then across your chest visualise two vibrant blue triangles intersecting in a mandala pointing upwards. Softly breathe in this Mandala with chanting the Bija Mantra YAM in your mind. Repeat this for 2 to 3 minutes.

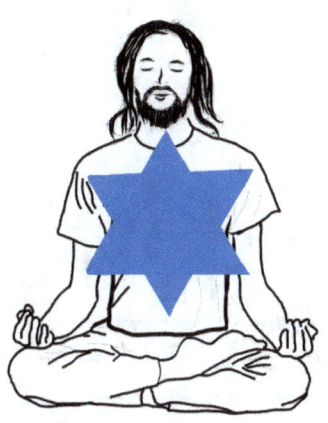

Mooladhara Chakra: Softly focus your mind at the base of your spine at the Mooladhara area and then gradually in the middle point and visualise a vibrant yellow square mandala across your root chakra area. Softly breathe in this Mandala by chanting the Bija Mantra LAM in your mind. Repeat this for 2 to 3 minutes.

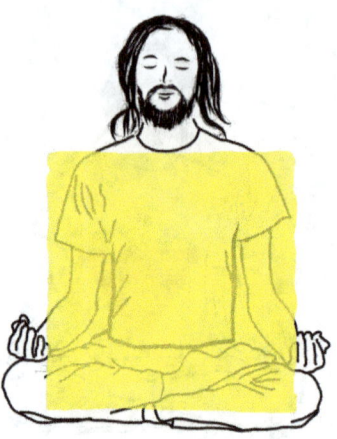

Vishuddha Chakra: Softly focus your mind across your throat area and then gradually in the middle point and visualise a vibrant oval magenta coloured mandala across your throat. Softly breath in this Mandala with chanting the Bija Mantra HAM in your mind. Repeat this for 2 to 3 minutes.

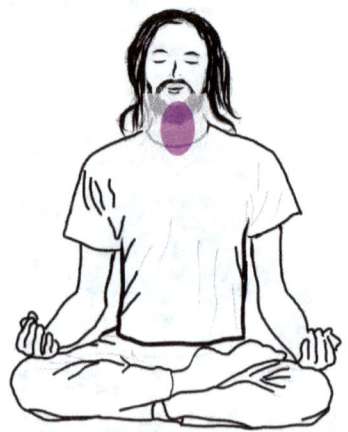

Ajna Chakra: Softly focus your mind across your third eye area and then gradually in the middle of the eyebrows and visualise a vibrant orange circle mandala across your third eye. Softly breathe in this Mandala with chanting the Bija Mantra ONG in your mind. Repeat this for 2 to 3 minutes.

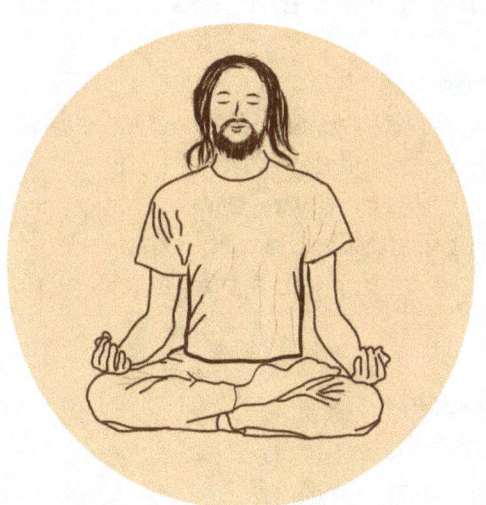

Sahashrara Chakra: Softly focus your mind at the top of your head or crown and then gradually in the middle point and visualise peace and silence expanding across your crown. Softly breathe in this Mandala with chanting the Bija Mantra OM in your mind. Repeat this for 2 to 3 minutes.

Pancha-Mahabhutas in Summary

Pancha Mahabhutas
1. Akasha provides spaciousness which 'allows' for movement
2. Vayu provides the driving force behind all movement
3. Agni provides energy for transformation and illumination
4. Jala is lubricating, and provides moisture, flow and cooling
5. Prithvi provides structure, form and stability

Qualities of Akasha:
-minute (very small)
-light
-soft
-smooth

Functions of Akasha:
-vastness
-expansive
-all-compassing
-all-accommodating

Qualities of Vayu:
-Light
-Cold
-Rough
-Coarse
-Non-slimy

Functions of Vayu:
- movement
- roughness
- reduction

- lightness
- non-sliminess

Qualities Of Agni:
– Hot
– Sharp
– Minute
– Light
– Rough
– Non-slimy

Functions Of Agni:
- Heat
- Digestion
- Lustre
- Light
- Complexion

Qualities Of Jala:
– Light
– Unctuous
– Cold
– Dull
– Soft
– Slimy

Functions Of Jala:

- Moistening
- Lubricating
- Binding
- Oozing
- Softening

- Exhilarating CSF
- Saliva
- Plasma/Pericardial fluid
- Pleural fluid
- Gastric juices
- ultrafiltrate of plasma/urine
- Intracellular fluid/cytoplasm

Qualities Of Prithvi:
– Heavy
– Coarse
– Hard
– Dull
– Stable
– Non-slimy
– Solid
– Gross

Functions Of Prithvi:
– Development
– Compactness
– Heaviness
– Firmness

Relation of Bhutas And Energy

Relation Of Bhutas and Energy

Element	Energy
Space	Sound
Fire	Solar
Air	Wind
Water	Rain
Earth	Gravitational & Magnetic force

Deity of Bhutas

Deity of Bhutas

Prithvi - goddess Bhūdevi & Brahma.
Jala – Varuṇa & Vishṇu
Vayu– Vayu Deva & Hanuman
Agni - Agni Deva & Shiva
Akasha – Parameshvara or Sadashiva which is all pervading

Gunas and Bhutas:

Bhuta	Guna
Akasha	Satva Dominant
Agni	Satva and Rajas Dominant
Vayu	Rajas dominant
Jala	Sattva and Tamas dominant
Prithvi	Tamas dominant

Characteristics of Pancha-Mahabhuta

Bhuta	Characteristics
Akasha	Free flow/unobstructability (Apratighatata)
Agni	Heat (Ushnatva)
Vayu	Mobility (Chalatva)
Jala	Liquidity (Dravatva)
Prithvi	Roughness (Kharatva)

Key Mantras for Pancha Mahabhutas

1. Tasmadva etasmadatmana akash sambhutah |
Akasadvayuh | Vayoragnih | Agnerapah |
Adbhyah prithvi | Prithivya osadhayah |
Osadhibhyosnam |Annat purusah ||

Meaning: From that atman (Supreme Self) Akasha manifests, From Vayu manifests from Akasha, from Vayu manifests Agni, from Agni manifests Jala, and from Jala manifests Prathvi. From Prithvi we receive plants, from plants come food and from food human being's manifest.
Source: "Yajurveda, Taittiriyopanisad"

Agni Gayatri Mantra:-

   Om Maha-jwalaya Vidamahe Agni Madhyaya Dhimahi |

   Tanno Agnih Prachodayate Om||

Let me invoke and meditate on the great flame, Oh God of fire, bless me with the light of higher intellect, and let the Fire God illuminate my mind.

Varun / Jal Gayatri Mantra:-

   Om Jala bimbhaya Vidamahe Nila Purushaya Dheemahi !

   Tanno Varuna Prachodayate Om !

Let me invoke and meditate on the reflection of water, Oh God of ocean blue, bless me with coolness of higher intellect, and let the God of water illuminate my mind.

Vayu Gayatri Mantra:-

Om pawan-purushaya vidamahe sahstramurtiye ch dhimhi !

Tanno vayuh prachodayate Om !

Let me invoke and meditate on the life-giving God of air. One who holds the sceptre, bless me with higher intellect, and let the God of Winds illuminate my mind.

Akasha Gayatri Mantra:-

Om Akashaya cha Vidamahe Nabho Devaya Dheemahi !

Tanno Gaganam Prachodayate Om!

Let us invoke and meditate on the God of the Ethereal realm of skies, bless me with higher intellect, and let the Akasha God illuminate my mind.

Prithvi Gayatri Mantra:-

Om Vasundharaya Vidamahe Bhuta-dhatraya Dhimahi !

Tanno Bhumih Prachodayate Om !

Let us invoke and meditate on Bhumi Devi, The One who provides all that we need, bless us with abundance and let the Earth Goddess illuminate my mind.

Asanas, Kriyas and Pranayama for Pancha-Bhutas

Asanas for Prithvi Suddhi
(Perform following postures, holding them for 2 to 3 minutes)

1.   Baddha Konasana – Sit straight with soles of your feet joined together and heels close to the yoni nadi. Gently press your knees down towards floor and clasp both feet inside both the hands with fingers interlaced.

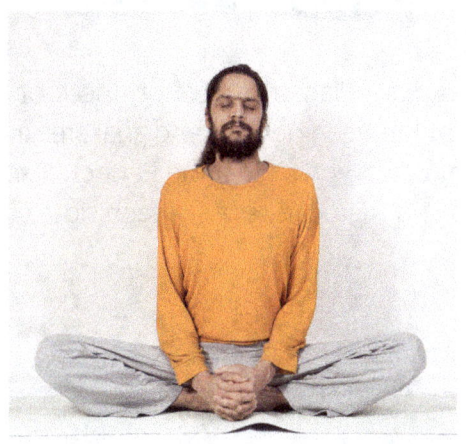

2.   Padmasana – Place the right foot on top of the left thing and left foot on top of the right thigh to Perform Lotus Pose. Hold your posture with Jnana Mudra. Practice on each side for 2 to 3 minutes.

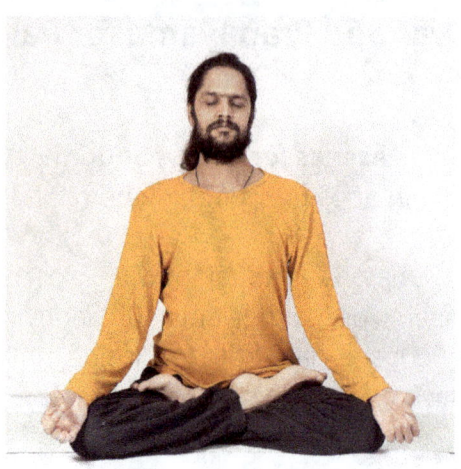

3. Siddhasana – Place the heel of one foot against the Yoni Nadi – the point between genitals and anal area and cover the foot with other foot on top of it. Hold the Perfect Pose with Dhyana or Jnana Mudra. Hold the postures with each side for 2 to 3 minutes.

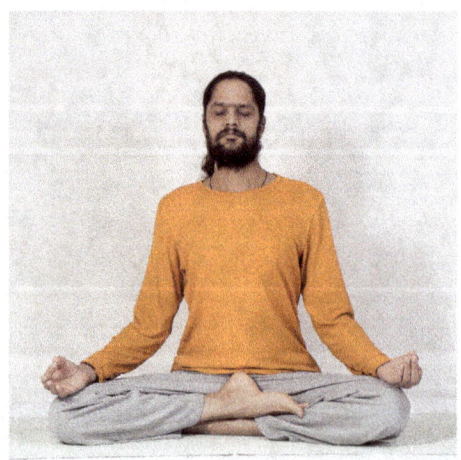

4. Veerasana – From standing with legs wide open, turn your right foot pointing away and extend your arms along both the shoulders. Bend your right knee to ninety-degree angle. Hold your posture for 2 to 3 minutes on each side.

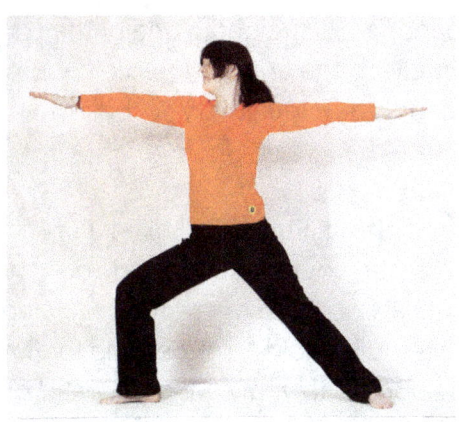

5.   Tittali Kriya - – Sit straight with soles of your feet joined together and heels close to the yoni nadi. Gently bounce your knees for 2 to 3 minutes.

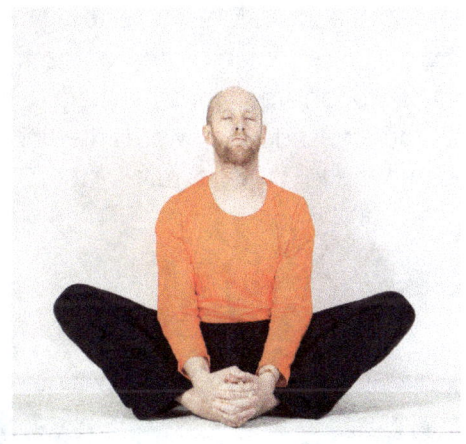

6. Moolabandha- Sit straight in one of the comfortable asana. Now squeeze or clinch the anal and pelvic floor muscles and hold on the moolabandha. Gradually try to build this Bandha upto 3 minutes.

Pranayama For Prithvi Suddhi: (Sukha Purvaka Pranayama) – Sit straight and focus your mind around root-chakra and follow 9 rounds of Sukha Purvaka Pranayama following the breathing pattern of -inhale for 8 x hold for 8 x exhale for 8 x hold for 8). The counting can be done with your own heart beats or ticking of clock.

Asanas for Jala Suddhi
(Perform following posture, holding them for 2 to 3 minutes)

1. Janu-sirasasana – Sit straight with one leg extended straight in front with the foot of other leg on top of the thigh. Gently fold forward to catch hold on your foot of straight leg and stretch forward to bring your chest down towards the thigh and chin over the knee of straight leg. Hold the posture for 2 to 3 minute on each side.

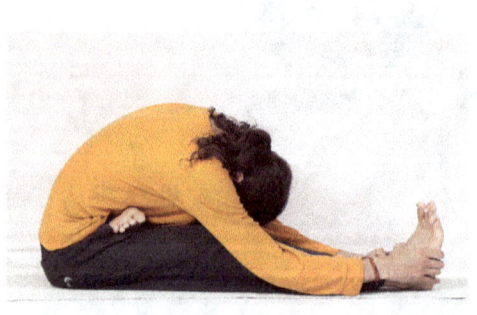
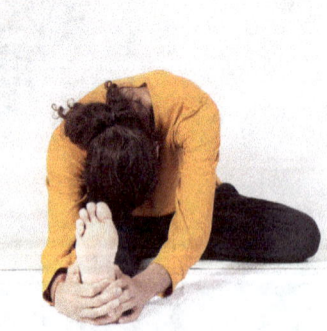

2.   Yoga Mudra – Come to Padmasana and reach your hands from behind to catch hold on to the big toes with arms crossing to opposite side.

3.   Eka and Dwi Pada Uttana Asana – Lay straight in. Shavasana and practice single leg lift and double leg life pose for 2 to 3 minutes.

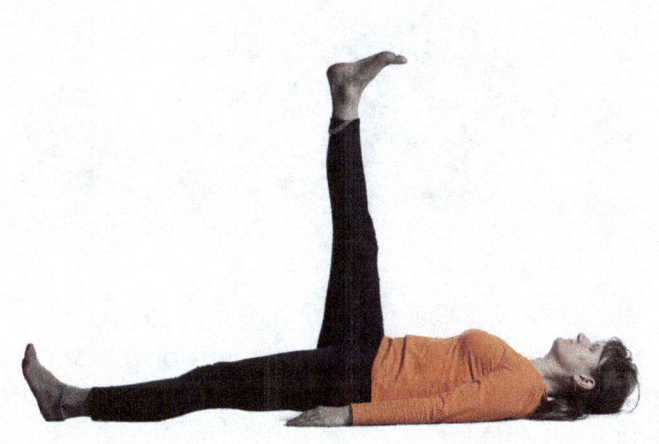

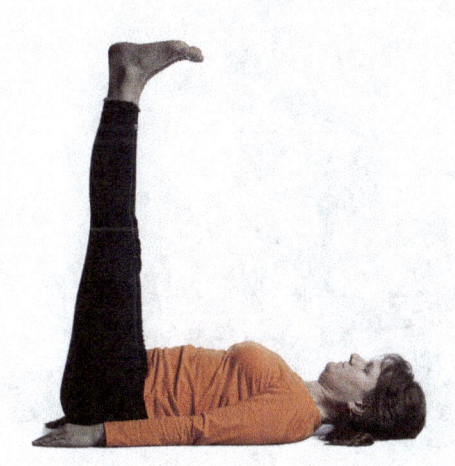

4. Kati-Chakra Asana and or Kriyas – Lay on your back with knees bend and heels on floor close to buttocks. Keep your arms straight along the shoulders on floor. Bring your knees on floor to right side and head to left to create a twist. Hold on the posture for 2 to 3 minutes on each side.

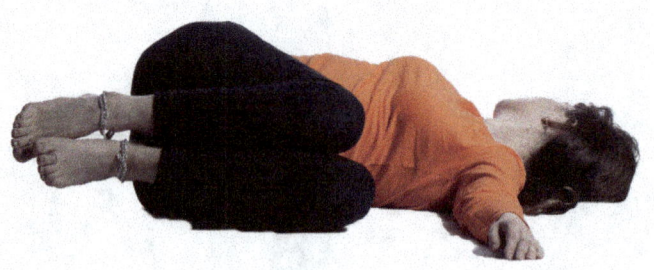

5. Maha Mudra – Place the right foot against the yoni nadi with keeping the left leg straight. Fold forward with catching hold of right foot to bring your chest over the thigh, chin over the knee and hold the posture for 2 to 3 minutes.

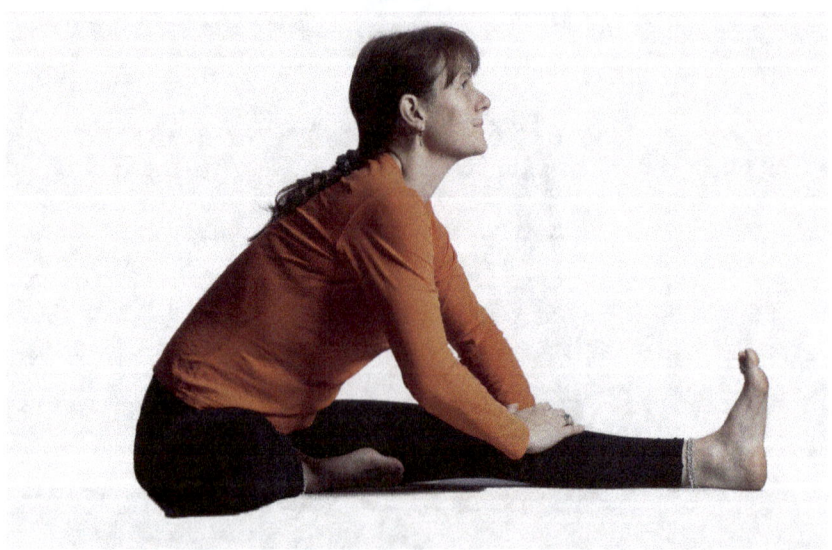

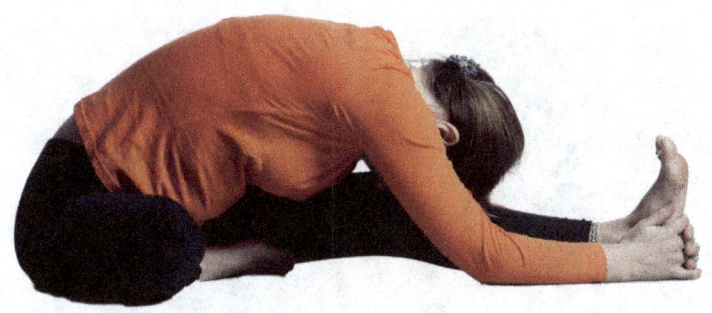

6. Ashwini Mudra – Sit in one of the cross-legged posture. Gently squeeze and clinch the anal muscles and let go and relax them. Perform this kriya for 2 to 3 minutes.

Pranayama for Jala Suddhi: (Sukha Vritti Pranayama) Sit straight and focus your mind around sacral area and follow 9 rounds of Sukha Vritti Pranayama following the breathing pattern of -inhale for 8 x exhale for 8. The counting can be done with your own heart beats or ticking of clock.

Asanas for Agni Suddhi
(Perform following posture, holding them for 2 to 3 minutes)

1.   Navasana Kriyas and Asana – Sit straight with both the legs to the front. With balancing on your sitting bones, raise both your legs up towards the front with keeping the arms extended along the legs towards the feet.

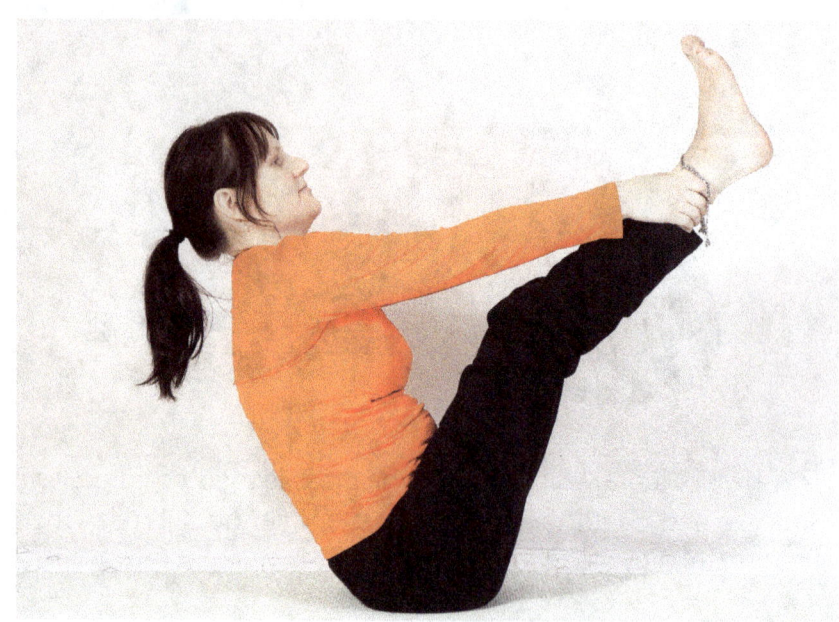

2.	Samtulasana – Balance on your straight arms and your toes with body suspended straight in plank position.

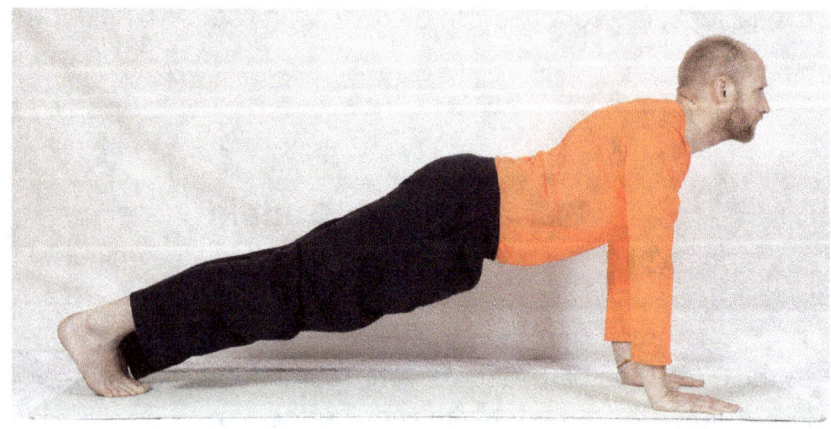

3.	Paschimottanasana – Sit straight with legs straight in front. Reach forward to catch hold to your feet, draw your chest over to the thighs and chin towards the knees. Hold the posture for 2 to 3 minutes.

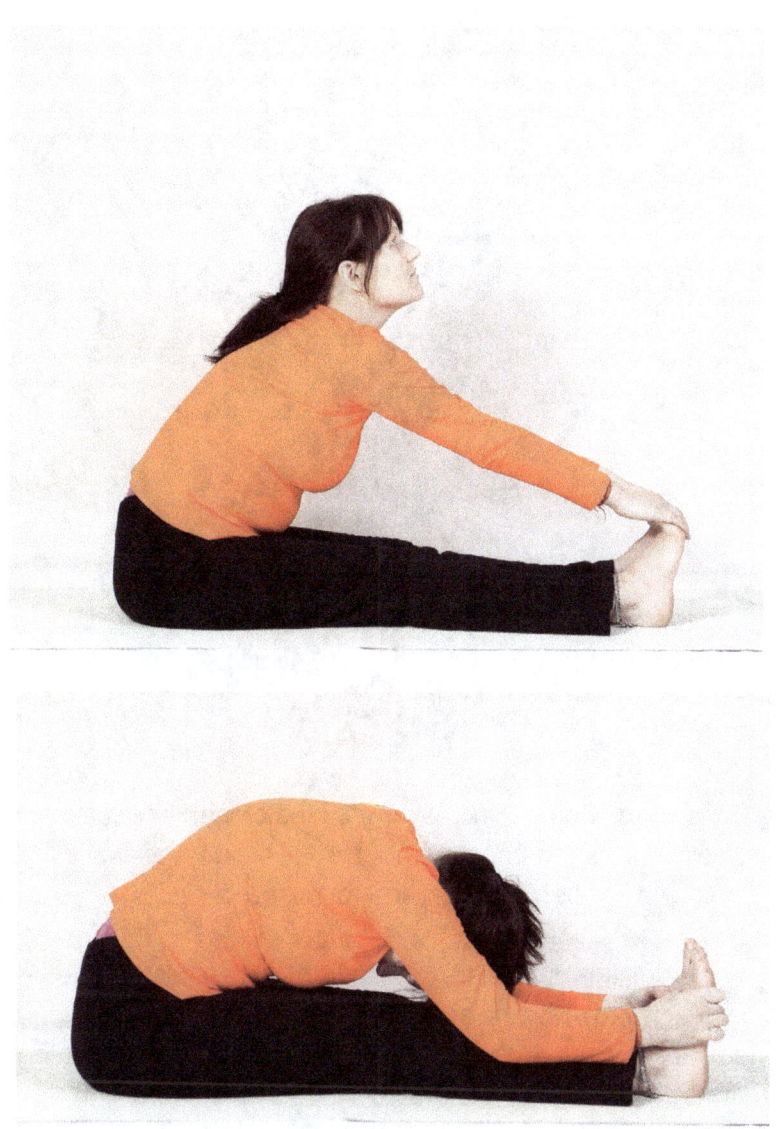

4.   Viparita Karni Mudra – From Shavasana come to double leg lift (Dwi-Pada-Uttana-Asana). Gradually more up to Sarvanga Asana or shoulder stand. Now gently bring your feet slightly down to front as in image and hold the posture for 2 to 3 minutes.

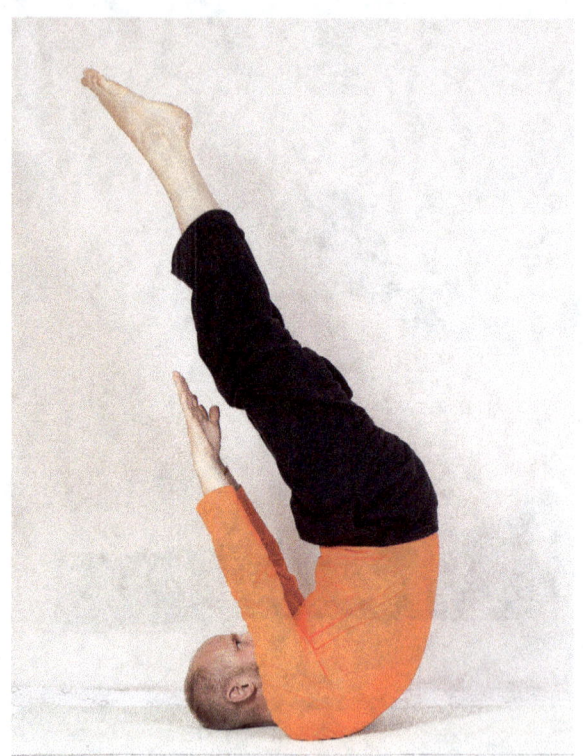

5.	Tadagi Mudra – In Shavasana inhale deep whilst expanding the belly. Hold the breath and try to create the waves whilst pumping the abdomen back, and forth and in circles.

6.	Uddiyana Bandha – Sit straight in a comfortable Asana. Exhale fully and draw the abdomen inward and upward to perform Unddiyan Bandha. Hold the 10 to 15 counts whilst holding the breath out. Repeat it 3 to 5 times.

Pranayama for Agni Suddhi: (Loma Vritti Pranayama) Sit straight and focus your mind around stomach area and follow 9 rounds of Loma-Vritti Pranayama following the breathing pattern of -inhale for 8 x hold in for 8 x exhale for 8. The counting can be done with your own heart beats or ticking of clock.

Asanas for Vayu Suddhi
(Perform following posture, holding them for 2 to 3 minutes)

1.   Ustrasana – From Vajrasana come to kneeling position, bend back to reach your hands on your heals, to stretch your back and open the heart area. Hold the posture for 2 to 3 minutes.

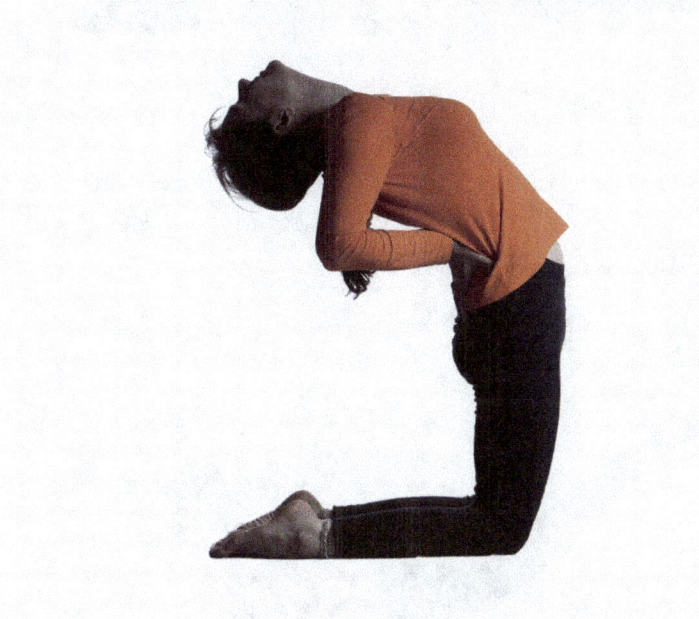

2.   Matsyasana – Lay in Sukhasana or Padmasana. With the support of your elbows raise your chest up whilst coming up on top of back of head. Finally reach your hands to touch on your thighs or catch on toes whilst keeping the elbows on floor.

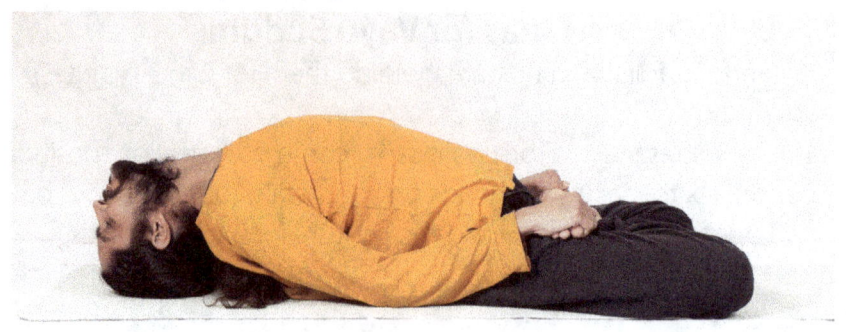

3. Shalbha and Chiri Kriya –

3.1 Shalbha Kriya – Come to four-footed pose. Raise your one leg behind whilst inhalation and bring it back down whilst exhalation. Repeat it three times with each leg.

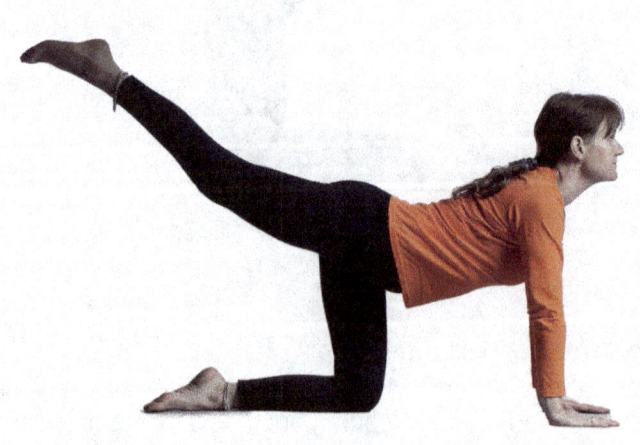

3.2. Chiri Kriya – Whilst inhalation raise your one leg behind and whilst exhalation draw your head and knee together. Repeat 3 times with each leg.

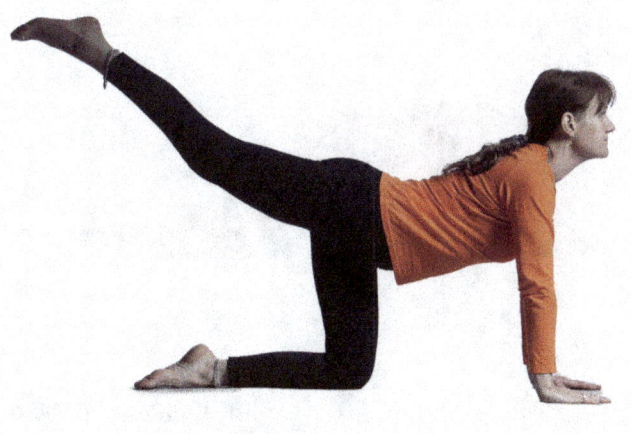

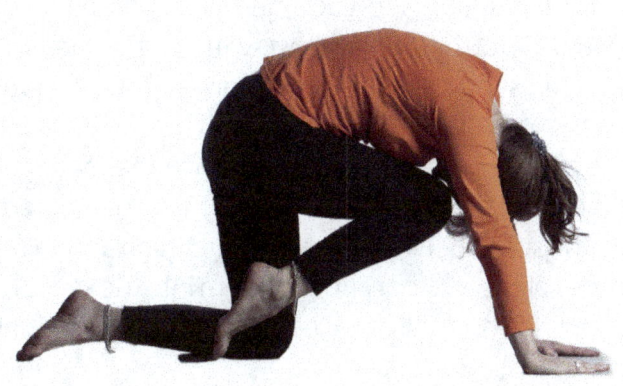

4. Sasanga Asana- From Vajrasana place both your hands on floor in front of the knees whilst keeping the arms straight and forehead on the floor. Gently push your chest forward and follow 2 to 3 minutes conscious mid-chest breathing.

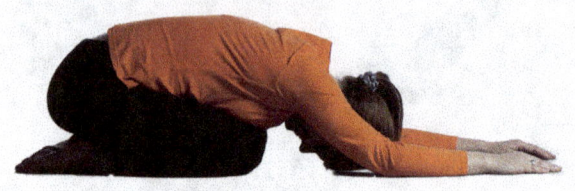

5.	Nikunja Asana - Sit straight in vajrasana. Slowly move your chest and hands forward, lifting up the hips without moving the knees and feet from their position and place the right side of your head on the ground. Your face should be facing the left side. Your upper chest should also be firmly placed to the ground. Try to keep your buttocks high and abdomen pushing downward. Now breathe deeply into the upper chest, with total awareness in the upper chest and shoulder area. Do the same on the opposite side.

6.	Swastikasana - Bend one leg to place the foot against the inside of the opposite thigh. Now, bend the other leg and place that foot in the space between the opposite thigh and calf muscles. Catch the toes of the first foot and pull them into the space between the opposite thigh and calf muscles. Sit straight in Jnana or Dhyana Mudra for 2 to 3 minutes.

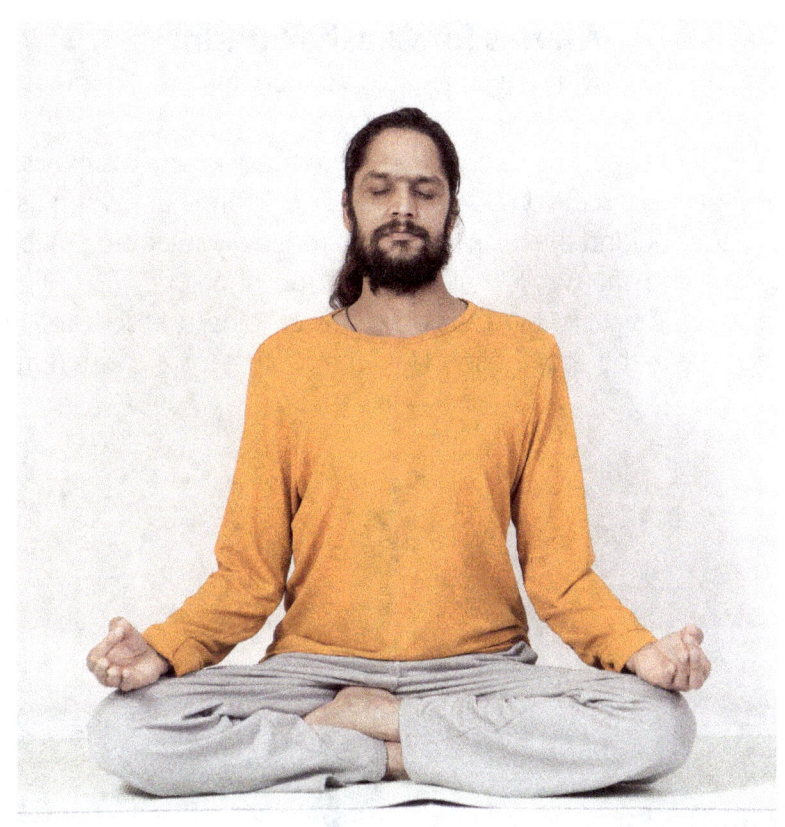

Pranayama for Vayu Suddhi: (Viloma Vritti Pranayama) (Inhale for 8 x exhale for 8x hold out for 8) Sit straight and focus your mind around the heart area and follow 9 rounds of Viloma Vritti Pranayama following the breathing pattern of -inhale for 8 x exhale for 8 x hold out for 8. The counting can be done with your own heart beats or ticking of clock.

Asanas for Akasha Suddhi

(Perform following posture, holding them for 2 to 3 minutes)

1.   Sarvangasana - Slowly come into the dvi-pada-uttana-asana on an in breath. Lift you're your legs, buttocks and back whilst using the hands behind the back to support to. Slowly straighten up both the legs and back whilst balancing on your shoulders. Try to lift up the legs and back as high as possible. Your spine, buttocks and legs should be in the straight line. Hold the posture for 2 to 3 minutes.

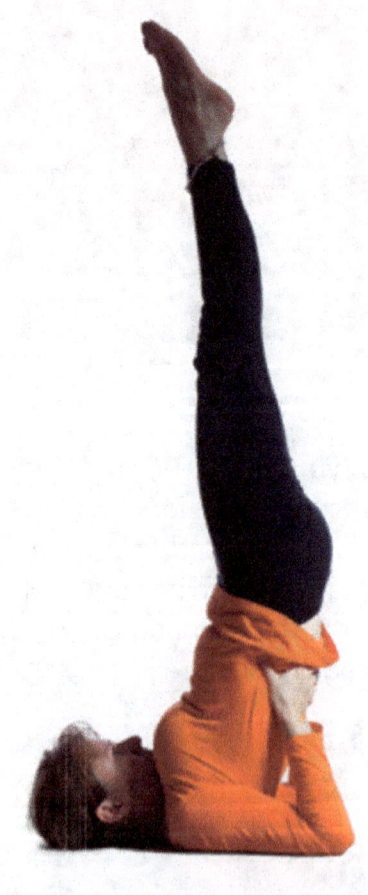

2. Setu-Bandhasana – Come to shavasana and then fold both your legs to place the heels against the buttocks. Place both the hands close to the feet or catch hold on to your heels or legs if possible. Now lift your buttcoks and back up with pushing the chest up by using the force of the hands. In Setu-Bandha Asana you can perform various hand mudras whilst holding the posture for 2 to 3 minutes.

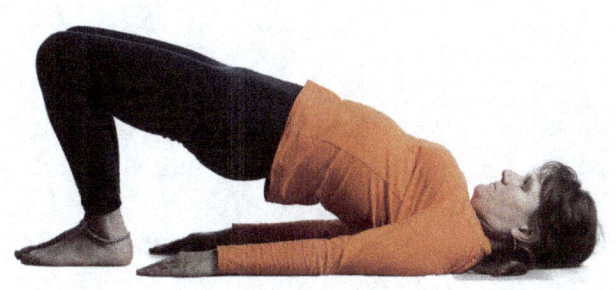

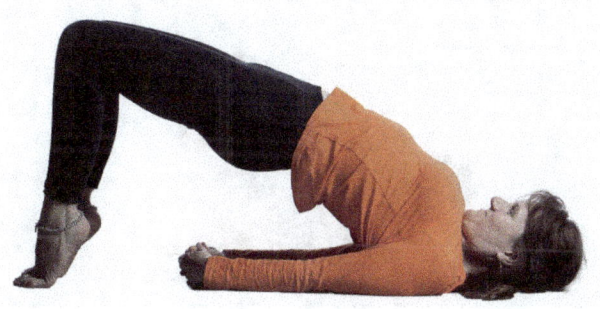

3. Sasanga Asana Paripurna- From Vajrasana fold forward to bring your head close to the knees in Dharmika Asana. Keep holding on your feet and raise your buttocks up whilst rolling on top of your head. Hold your posture for 2 to 3 minutes.

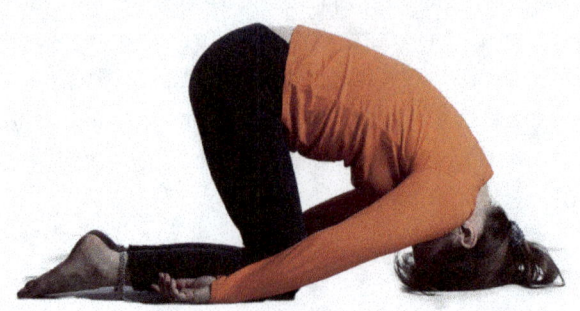

4. Halasana - Slowly from Shavasana come into the dvi-pada-uttana-asana on an in breath. Lift your buttocks and try to lift the legs behind the head to place the toes on the ground with keeping the spine straight and back high without folding the legs. Hold Halasana for 2 to 3 minutes.

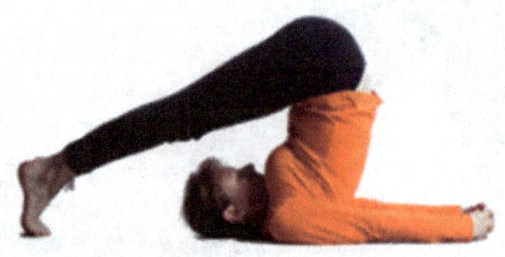

5. Jalandhara Bandha – Sit straight in one of the comfortable Asana. Gently press your chin down against the chest to perform the throat lock or Jalandhara Bandha. Hold this Bandha for 2 to 3 minutes.

Pranayama for Akasha Suddhi: (Ujjayi Pranayama) – Sit straight in a comfortable Asana. Inhale and exhale gently whilst making the sound of breath by contracting the back of throat. Follow 9 rounds of Ujjayi Pranayama.

Asanas for Pancha-Mahabhuta Suddhi
(Perform following posture, holding them for 2 to 3 minutes)

1. Dharmika Asana followed by Vajrasana Supta

1.1. Dharmika Asana – In Vajrasana fold forward to place your top of forehead close to the knees whilst arms reaching behind to touch the soles of feet. Hold this asanas with focussing the mind at Jyoti-Bindu at top of your forehead.

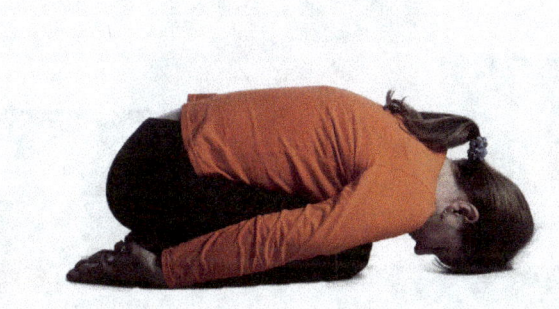

1.2. Vajrasana Supta – Return back to Vajrasana and recline back to place back of your head on floor whilst hands touching on top of thighs and elbows on floor. Hold the posture for 2 to 3 minutes whilst visualising the light at top of your crown or Brahmarandra Bindu.

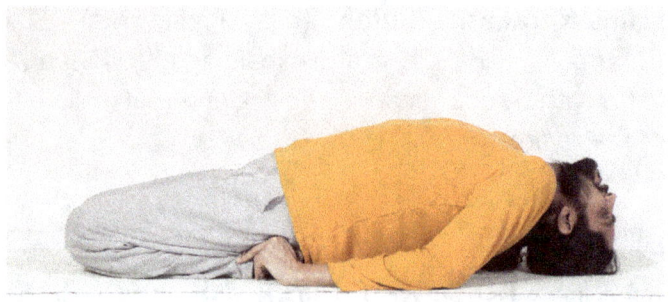

2. Paschimottanasana, Navasana, Dwipadauttanasana, Sarvangasana, Halasana
    1.1. Paschimottanasana
    1.2. Navasana
    1.3. Dwipadauttanasana
    1.4. Sarvangasana
    1.5. Halasana

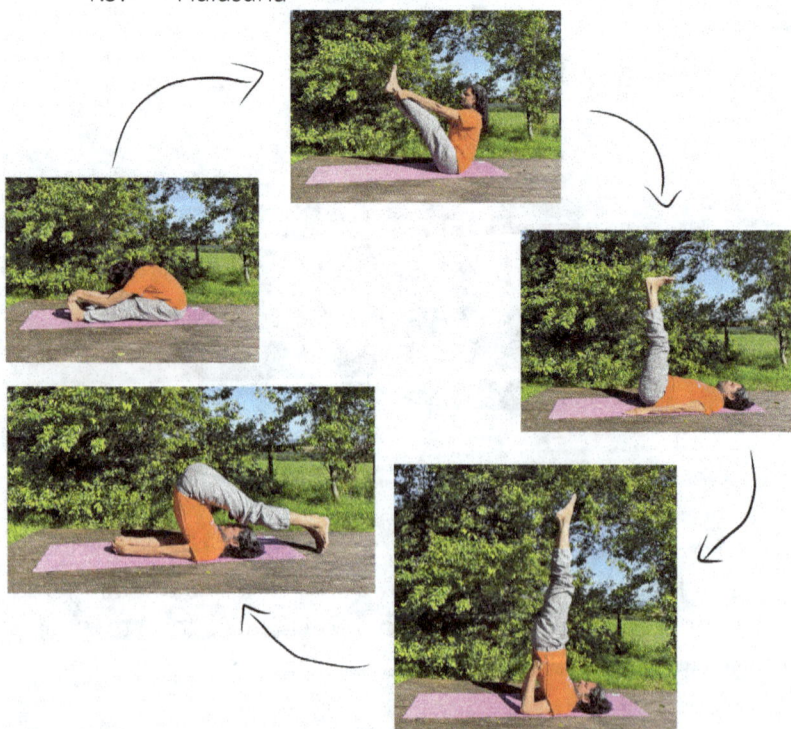

3.   Chakrasana - Lye on floor with feet on floor close to buttocks and knees pointing to ceiling. Now place your hands on floor over your shoulders and fingers pointing back to shoulders. Slowly lift your body up to balance on your arms and legs. Hold your posture for few conscious breaths to gradually hold for 2 to 3 minutes.

4.   Shirasasna - From Vajrasana place both your hands on floor and interlace your fingers. Now open you elbows to create a nice tripod to balance. Place top of your head on floor close to your clasped hands. Now slowly raise both your legs straight over to ceiling with maintaining the balance on your crown and tripod of hands. Hold it for few breaths.

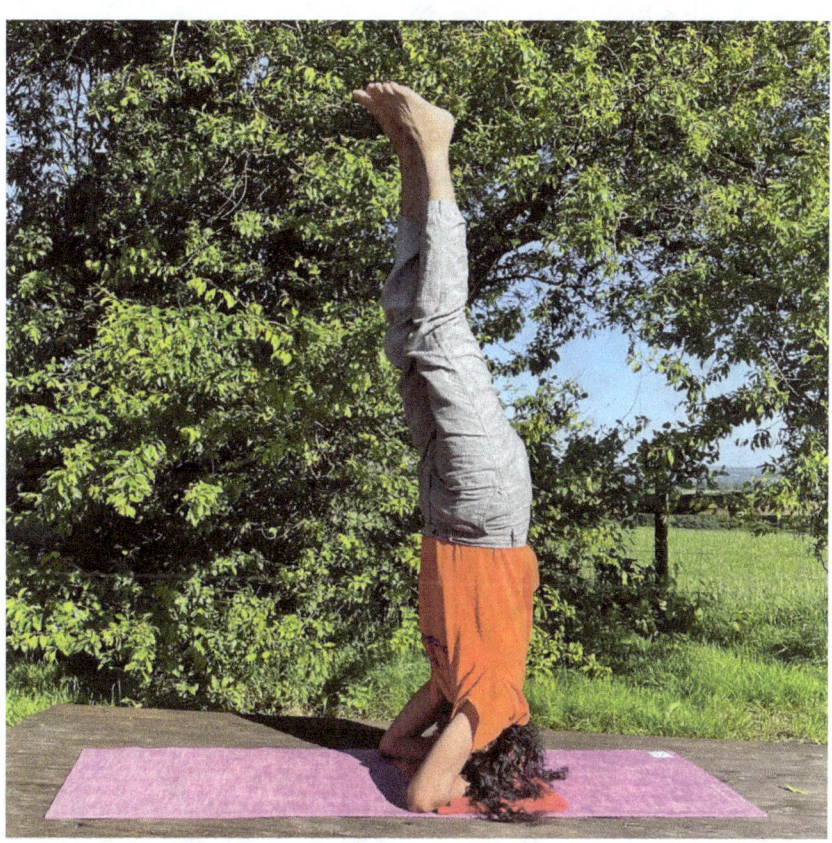

5. Padmasana, Baddhapadmasana, Yogamudra, Matsyasana, Gupta-Padmasana.

5.1. Padmasana
5.2. Baddhapadmasana- From Padmasana cross both your hands behind to catch hold on toes of your feet.
5.3. Yoga Mudrasana –From Baddha-Padmasana gently fold forward to place your forehead on floor and hold your posture for 2 to 3 minutes.
5.4. Matsyasana – Lay on your back in Padmasana. With the support of your elbows along both sides, lift your chest and shoulders up to balance on top of back of the head.
5.5. Gupata-Padmasana – Lay on face-prone position in Padmasana with hands behind the heart in Hamsa Mudra.

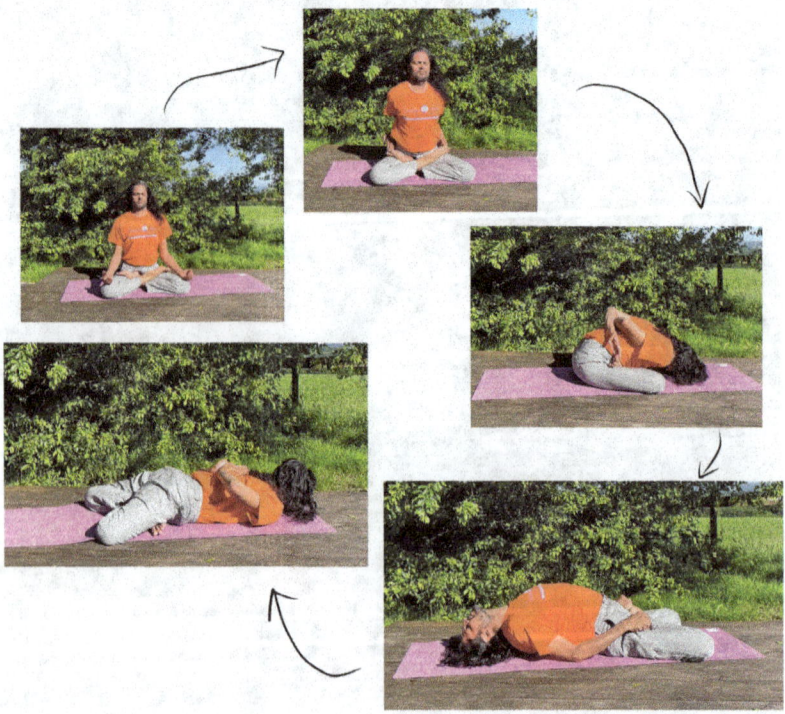

6.   Raja-Kapota Asana – From four-footed position, bring your left knee on floor between your hands whilst keeping the right leg straight. Now fold your right leg with foot pointing back towards head. Place your right hand behind that foot so you can hold your foot in side the elbow and point your right hand back towards head. Gradually lift your left arm over your head and reach back to catch hold of your right hand.

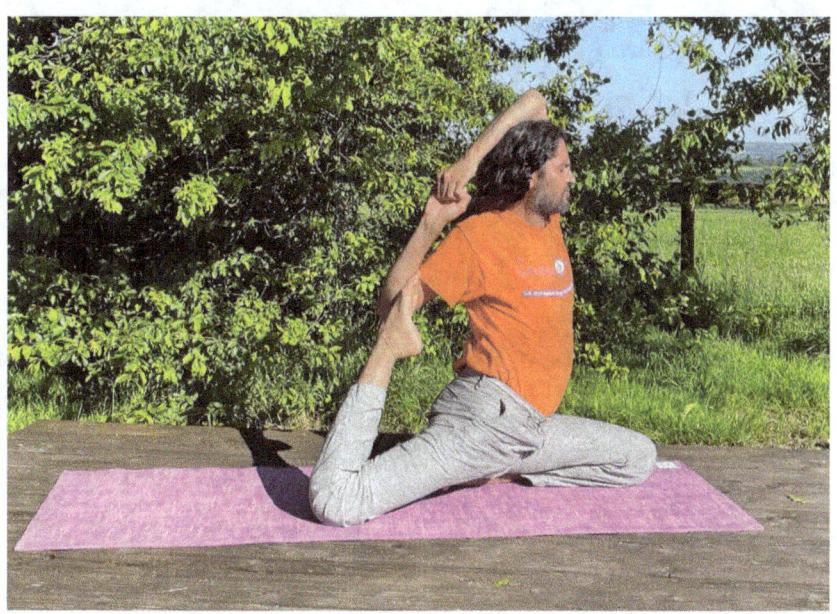

7.   Dhanurasana – Lay on face-prone position. Fold both your legs to catch hold on your feet or ankle joints. Raise your head, chest and legs in the stretch to balance on your abdominal area.

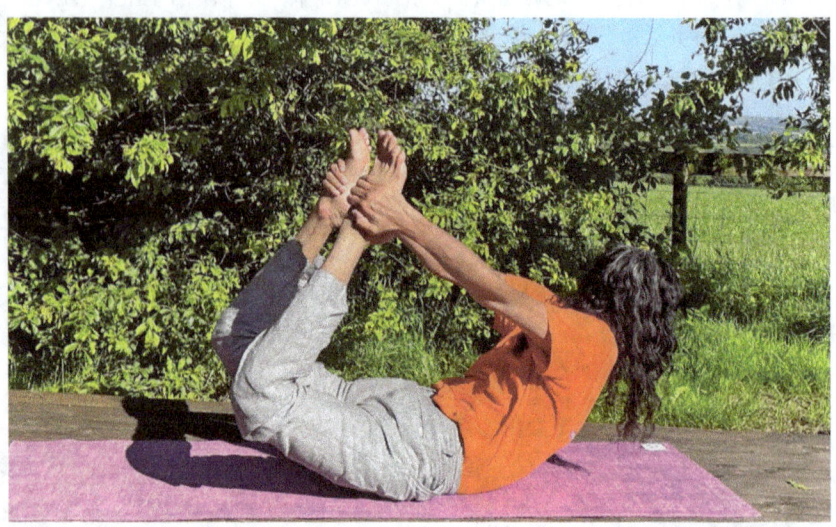

8.   Mahabhuta-Mudras – Hold mahabhuta mudras for a minute in a comfortable posture.
      8.1.   Prathvi Mudra
      8.2.   Jala or Varuna Mudra
      8.3.   Vayu Mudra
      8.4.   Agni or Surya Mudra
      8.5.   Akasha Mudra

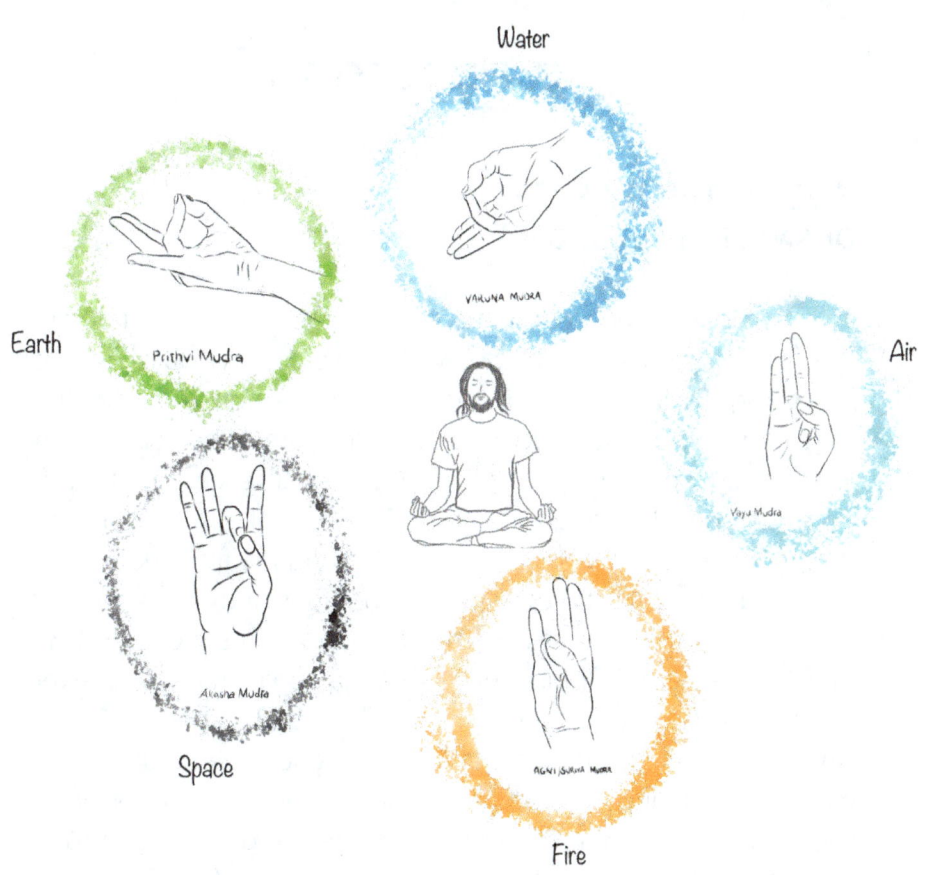

9. Mahabandha – Sit straight in one of the comfortable Dhyana-Asana. Exhale out your breath and whilst holding the breath out, hold all three Bandhas together for 10-15 counts. Repeat this 3 times.

Pranayama for Pancha-Mahabhuta Suddhi: Nadi Suddhi and Anuloma-Viloma Pranayama.

KEY RESOURCES

YOGA: STEP-BY-STEP
Dr. Swami Gitananda Giri

This correspondence course is one of the best basic training in Classical Yoga through the written word now available. The Yoga: Step-By-Step Correspondence Course study is one of the requirements for those desiring to participate in the Six Month International Yoga Teacher's Training Course held each year at ICYER from October 2 through March 25th. Yogamaharishi Dr. Swami Gitananda developed this course in 1971 and the fifty-two weekly lessons are well illustrated with photographs and line drawings. It contains a practical, systematic step-by-step instruction in the integral practice of Rishiculture Ashtanga Yoga. Students answer the weekly lesson-questionnaire and submit their papers to ICYER - Ananda Ashram for evaluation. Correspondence. The Guru carefully goes through all papers and establishes a personal rapport with the students, through regular correspondence guiding each one through problems and difficulties. A Certificate of proficiency is awarded upon successful completion of the course. Included, as a bonus is a free three-year subscription to the monthly journal Yoga Life.

PRANAYAMA IN THE TRADITION OF RISHICULTURE ASHTANGA YOGA:
Dr. Swami Gitananda Giri, Yogacharini Meenakshi Devi Bhavanani and Dr. Ananda Balayogi Bhavanani

Various essays on Pranayama in the Rishiculture Ashtanga Yoga tradition have been condensed into this book. It offers a study of not only the classical eight Pranayamas but also gives a brief understanding of the 120 Pranayamas as taught by Dr Swami Gitananda Giri. A must for any sincere student of wanting to expand their knowledge of Pranayama.

CHAKRAS: THE PSYCHIC CENTRES OF YOGA AND TANTRA
Dr. Ananda Balayogi Bhavanani

According to the Rishiculture Ashtanga Yoga tradition codified by Yogamaharishi Dr Swami Gitananda Giri, there are six lower and six higher Chakras making a total of twelve Chakras. The lower Chakras known as the Pinda Chakras are related to the physical body while the higher six Chakras, the Anda Chakras are related to the Cosmos. Chakras vibrate at very high speeds of vibration and at their highest speeds of vibration are related to the cosmos. Each of the lower six Chakras has various neuro-endocrine correlates and is associated with one of the five Jnanendriyas and Karmendriyas as also different psychological qualities. This book deals with the Chakras in a detailed manner with magnificent images that were conceptualized by Pujya Swamiji more than 50 years ago. Asanas related to each Chakra and their specific Mandala Pranayamas are elaborated in detail. The unique practices of Chakra Mediation and Mandala Dharana are also added bonuses in this book.

MUDRAS (New Edition)
Dr. Swami Gitananda Giri

This is a completely revised and upgraded edition of the original book by the great Yogamaharishi. A good deal of material is available to the modern student on the subject of Hatha Yoga Asanas, Shat Karmas and a bit on Pranayama. Little is however found when searching for information on Mudras that represent some of the deeper practices of the Yoga system. Mudra is the ancient Yogic art and science of gesturing and sealing vital Pranic energies in the human body for health, well being and spiritual evolution. These are advanced techniques designed to improve neuromuscular coordination, culture human emotions and still the restless mind. In Yoga and Tantra, Mudras are used with the most evolutionary knowledge available to the serious student about the relationship between energy flows in the tissues, nerve channels and organs of the body as well as their correlation to higher flows of Prana in the subtle and causal bodies. In the higher practices of Yoga, Mudras are used to "gesture" the mind, Prana and the lower and higher Shaktis through the Nadis, or subtle nerve channels of the Pancha Kosha, the Five Bodies of Man. A short practice of the Prana Mudras will soon convince even the most skeptical student of their value. The Oli Mudras are amongst the most valuable techniques to be undertaken by a serious student of Yoga. The Shakti Mudras represent the highest form of sublimation of lower energy drives into the bountiful Ojas and Tejas, the higher forces produced in the human body by the Yogis.

HATHA YOGA PRACTICES OF THE RISHICULTURE ASHTANGA YOGA TRADITION
Dr. Ananda Balayogi Bhavanani

This book by Dr Ananda Balayogi Bhavanani is intended for the intelligent, philosophically-minded Sadhaka or Seeker of Truth who is not only seeking excellence in his/her or her profession, but is also seeking to live a full well-rounded, humane and elevated life. It is clearly laid out with instruction given in basic Asanas, Kriyas, Mudras and Pranayama of Gitananda Yoga (Rishiculture Ashtanga Yoga), along with explanations of their benefits and uses. A syllabus of instruction for 30 graded lessons is also provided at the end to enable the fuller understanding for both the teacher and student alike. Comments are also made on the role of healthy diet and relaxation in the well-rounded life. Interesting insights are offered into the body's glandular system, and the role of Yoga practice in its stimulation. This book is a useful practical instruction manual for Yoga teachers in educational institutions and can provide guidelines for Physical Education teachers desirous of adding Yoga practices to their curriculum. The material in this book is useful to seekers from all walks of life as it provides a clear and basic, step-by-step instruction to elementary Hatha Yoga concepts and practices of Gitananda Yoga. This book contains a few of the "sets or routine" that have been systematized in the Rishiculture Ashtanga Yoga tradition to produce particular results. The first "set" or routine detailed is the "Samasthiti Series" that is a set of Asanas designed to produce strength, flexibility, endurance, balance and stamina of the whole body. The second set or routine described in detail are the "Hathenas" that are designed to produce a powerful respiratory system preventing and controlling many respiratory disorders that are common in today's world. The third set of practices is of those belonging to the "Loma Viloma Series" that are designed to relieve neurasthenia and restore vital energy to a debilitated nervous system. They provide balanced energy flows for a debilitated nervous system thus energizing the whole being as well as providing a gentle stimulus to the spine, the digestive system, and all organs of the abdominal and pelvic cavities.

HATHA YOGA PRACTICES OF THE RISHICULTURE ASHTANGA YOGA TRADITION
Dr. Ananda Balayogi Bhavanani

This book by Dr Ananda Balayogi Bhavanani is intended for the intelligent, philosophically-minded Sadhaka or Seeker of Truth who is not only seeking excellence in his/her or her profession, but is also seeking to live a full well-rounded, humane and elevated life. It is clearly laid out with instruction given in basic Asanas, Kriyas, Mudras and Pranayama of Gitananda Yoga (Rishiculture Ashtanga Yoga), along with explanations of their benefits and uses. A syllabus of instruction for 30 graded lessons is also provided at the end to enable the fuller understanding for both the teacher and student alike. Comments are also made on the role of healthy diet and relaxation in the well-rounded life. Interesting insights are offered into the body's glandular system, and the role of Yoga practice in its stimulation. This book is a useful practical instruction manual for Yoga teachers in educational institutions and can provide guidelines for Physical Education teachers desirous of adding Yoga practices to their curriculum. The material in this book is useful to seekers from all walks of life as it provides a clear and basic, step-by-step instruction to elementary Hatha Yoga concepts and practices of Gitananda Yoga. This book contains a few of the "sets or routine" that have been systematized in the Rishiculture Ashtanga Yoga tradition to produce particular results. The first "set" or routine detailed is the "Samasthiti Series" that is a set of Asanas designed to produce strength, flexibility, endurance, balance and stamina of the whole body. The second set or routine described in detail are the "Hathenas" that are designed to produce a powerful respiratory system preventing and controlling many respiratory disorders that are common in today's world. The third set of practices is of those belonging to the "Loma Viloma Series" that are designed to relieve neurasthenia and restore vital energy to a debilitated nervous system. They provide balanced energy flows for a debilitated nervous system thus energizing the whole being as well as providing a gentle stimulus to the spine, the digestive system, and all organs of the abdominal and pelvic cavities.

CLASSICAL HATHA YOGA: 84 CLASSICAL ASANAS AND THEIR VARIATIONS
Yogachariya Jnandev Giri

In Shiva Samhita, Hatha Yoga Pradipika, Gheranda Samhita and other scriptures there is mention of 8,400,000 Asanas, which means form of births or life, YONI. We all have to go through each and every life form to learn and experience to grow. Out of those they say only 84 are important. Out of those 84 only 32 are most important and out of those, 4 sitting postures are essential ones. To be successful in pranayama and meditation one needs to master one of them. This book attempts to describe these 84 important postures as they were taught to me (Yogachariya Jnandev / Surender Saini).

EXPLORING YOGA PHILOSOPHY: 121 AUTHENTIC YOGA LESSONS
Yogachariya Jnandev Giri

This book is a compilation of knowledge acquired through several years deep study and immersion into the esoteric and philosophical sides of Yoga. Yoga is of course a full time activity when we understand it properly and it is one if the subjects that as we study it reveals more and more to us, an endless study of our own true innermost nature.
This book is aimed at Yoga Sadhaks practitioners who are embracing the yogic lifestyle and who want to sincerely study Yoga at it roots and grow and evolve spiritually as Human beings, evolving into higher thought and practices of Yoga.

SWARA YOGA
Yogachariya Jnandev Giri and Dr Ananda Balayogi Bhavanani

The Swara Yoga teachings come from "Shiva Swarodaya," an ancient Sanskrit Tantric text. This scripture or teachings are in the form of a dialogue between Lord Shiva and his wife Parvati. The text describes that Swara Yoga is useful for the transformation of our life and knowing how to perform various life activities based on breath, nostril and energy.

References: -

1. https://vedapulse.com/pancha-maha-bhuta
2. https://www.easyayurveda.com/2016/05/24/understanding-concept-panchamahabhuta-application-areas-utility-ayurveda-treatment/
3. https://en.wikipedia.org/wiki/Pancha_Bhoota
4. https://www.hinduwebsite.com/24principles.asp
5. Yoga Chikitsha By Dr Ananda Balayogi Bhavanani.
6. Yoga Step By Step by Swamiji Dr Gitananda Giriji.
7. Charaka Samhita with English Translation by R.K.Sharma & Bagawan Das Chowkamba Sanskrit series, Varanasi- 2001.
8. Vaisesika Darsana by Kanada,Nyayavishta mission Pub.Calcutta 1861
9. Ashtanga Samgraha-Ram Sastri Kinjavadekar- Chitrasala Press-Pune-1940 with commentary by Indu- Sutrastana.
10. https://healthyayurveda.com/panchamahabhutas-the-5-great-elements/
11. https://www.carakasamhitaonline.com/index.php/Pancha_mahabhuta
12. http://www.ayurvedaamritvani.com/pancha-mahabhutas---five-great-elements.html
13. https://www.yogapedia.com/definition/6892/pancha-mahabhuta
14. https://isha.sadhguru.org/global/en/wisdom/article/tips-to-cleanse-five-elements
15. https://www.carakasamhitaonline.com/mediawiki-1.32.1/index.php?title=Pancha_mahabhuta&mobileaction=toggle_view_mobile
16. https://gita-society.com/wp-content/uploads/PDF/108upanishads.pdf

Glossary

Sanskrita Terms	English Meaning
Adhyatma	Spirituality
Adhyatmic	Spiritual
Agni	Fire, Heat
Agni or Surya Mudra	Energy gesture to purify fire or energy element
Ahamkara	Ego
Ajna Chakra	Third Eye or Chakra of Will
Akasha	Space, voidness, ether
Akasha Mudra	Energy gesture to purify ether or space element
Ama	Toxins in our body
Anahata Chakra	Heart or Unstruck Chakra
Anamika	Ring finger
Anguli	Finger
Angustha	Thumb
Apas	Liquid, water
Apratighatatwa	Unobtructiveness
Artava	Female reproductive fluids
Asana	Posture, pose, pause, state of being
Asanga-Samgraha	A scripture or collection of teachings on Ayurveda
Ashram	A sacred space for spiritual teachings and practices
Ashta	Eight
Ashta-Prakriti	Eight primordial elements
Asthi Dhatu	Bones, cartilage
Asuddha	Impure
Atman	Soul, Individual Self
Avyakta	Unmanifested aspect
Ayurveda	Herbal medicine system of ancient India or Bharat-Varsha
Bharata-Varsha	Country of Bharata dynasty now known as India
Bhumi	Earth
Bhuta	Element
Bhuta Mudras	Energy gestures to purify the subtle elements

Bhuta Siddhi	Mastery of Elements
Bija	Seed
Bija Mantra	Sacred seed chants
Bindu	Point
Brahmande	Universe
Buddhi	discriminating, reasoning and causative intelligence
Buddhi-Tattva	Universal intellectual element
Chakra	Wheel, Subtle energy centre
Chalatwa	Mobility
Chetana	Consciousness
Darshana	Philosophy, life-view points
Dasha	Ten
Dharma	Duty, righteousness
Dhatus	Tissues or Body constitutes according to Ayurveda
Dhuna	Sacred fireplace in Ashrams
Dravatwa	Liquidity
Eka	One
Eka-dasha	Eleven
Ekadasa-Indriyas	Eleven faculties of experience including five cognitive, five action organs and mind
Gandha	Smell
Garbha	Womb
Gitananda Giriji	Founder of Gitananda Yoga
Granthis	Glands
Gurukula	Womb of Guru or Home of Guru where disciples can live, learn and follow spiritual practices in a safe environment
Hasta	Hand
Hatha Yoga	Physical practices including asana, mudra, pranayama and Shatkarmas for purifying the body, mind and subtle energy to prepare for spiritual practices
Hindu Darshana	Hindu Philosophy or way of living
Hiranya-Garbha	The golden womb of creative Mother Nature
Ishwara	Divine, God, Lord, Super Consciousness

Jala	Water
Jangam	Living or moving being
Jiva	Living Being
Jnana	Wisdom, Knowledge of Self
Jnana Yoga Kriyas	Yogic Visualisation
Kaniska	Little finger
Kappa Dosha	Fluid, lubrication
Karma	physical, mental, verbal and emotional actions
Karya-Dravya	Active products (Doshas)
Kharatwa	Solidity
Kshaya	Deterioration
Madhyama	Middle finger
Maha	Great, Subtle, Primordial
Mahat	Supreme Intellectual Principal
Majja Dhatu	Bone marrow, nerves
Mamsa Dhatu	Muscles
Manas	The mind
Mandala	Sacred geometric shapes
Manipuri Chakra	Solar Plexus, Precious life Jewel Chakra
Mantra	A sacred chant
Medda Dhatu	Fat
Mool	Basic, root, primary
Mooladhara Chakra	Root or Foundation Chakra
Mudra	Energy seal, Gesture
Naada	Sacred Sounds
Naada Bindu	Sacred Sound Centre
Nadis or Naris	Channels of subtle energy flow
Namaskar	Greeting, Salutation
Nitya	Eternal, continuous
OM	Divine or Cosmic Sound
Pachan	Digestion
Pachan Shakti	Digestive energy
Pancha	Five

Pancha-Jnanendriyas	Five sense organs of cognition
Pancha-Karmendriyas	Five organs of action
Pancha-Maha-Bhutan's	Five primary or constitutional elements
Pancha-Tanmatras	Five cognitive experiences
Parinam Siddhanta	Theory of universal evolution
Parinama	Result, Manifest, Outcome, evolution
Parmatman	Divine or Supreme Self
Pinde	Individual Body
Pitta Dosha	Fire, acidic nature
Prakriti	Nature, Manifestation Potential
Prakriti	Primordial Nature
Pramanuvad	Atomic theory
Prana	Vital life force
Prana Mudra	Energy gesture to purify Prana Vayu
Prana Vayu	Subtle energy current
Pranamaya Kesha	Subtle energy body or sheath
Pranava	Om, sound of divine
Pranayama	Subtle energy work by using breath as a tool
Prasara	Expansion
Prithivi	Earth, solid materials
Prithvi Mudra	Energy seal to purify earth element
Pujya	Respected one, one worthy of worshiping
Purusha	Individual Self, Soul
Rajas	Action
Rajasic Guna	The evolutionary or transformatory quality
Rakta Dhatu	Blood
Rasa	Taste
Rasa	Juice
Rasa Dhatu	Plasma
Rasa Siddhanta	Theory of six tastes
Rasa-Tanmatra	Object of taste
Rupa	Form, Shape, Beauty
Rupa-Tanmatra	Object of Vision

Sabda	Sound, word, vibration
Sabda-Guna-Visista	Special qualities of sound
Sadhu	Saint, renounced being
Samadhi	Union, Self-Realisation, Oneness
Samkhya Yoga	Analytical Yoga Philosophy
Saprsha-Tanmatra	Object of touch
Sattva	Purity, Equanimity
Sattvic Guna	The involuntary quality
Savitri	Solar
Sharira	Body
Shat	Six
Shat-Darshana	Six major Hindu philosophies or life-view points
Shatkarmas	Six cleansing practices
Shristi	Universe
Shukra	Male reproductive fluids
Siddhanta	Concept, Principle
Siddhi	Mastery, mystic powers
Sparsha	Touch
Sthavara	Non-living or non-moving
Sthula	Gross or Physical
Suddha	Pure
Suddhi	Purification
Sukshma	Subtle
Surya	Sun
Surya Namaskar	Sun salutation
Swadhisthana Chakra	Self-dwelling or sacral Chakra
Swamiji	Mastered Soul, All-Knowing
Tamas	Inertia
Tamasic Guna	Inertia or holding quality
Tarjani	Index finger
Tat	There
Tattvas	Elements
Teja	Energy, Heat, Life-force

Tri	Three
Tri-Dosha	Three primary qualities
Tri-Gunas	Three Modes of Nature
Upanishads	Hindu Scriptures, Simple explanation of complex Vedic teachings
Usnatwa	Hotness
Vaishasika Darshana	Life philosophy based on atomic theory of creation
Vardhaka	Enhancement or enhancing
Varuna Mudra	Energy gesture to purify water or liquid element
Vata Dosha	Wind
Vayu	Air
Vayu Mudra	Energy gesture to purify wind element
Vedas	Four Ancient Hindu Scriptures
Vijnana	Science
Vishuddha Chakra	Throat or Purity Chakra
Visista	Special, unique
Vriddhi	Aggravation
Vyakta	Manifested aspect
Vyapaka	All-pervading
Yat	Where
Yoga	Union, Oneness, Path, mean and goal
Yogacharini	One who teaches yoga by following yoga (female)
Yogachariya	One who teaches yoga by following yoga (male)
Yogic	Practices and attitude of Yoga

About Yogachariya Jnandev Giri (Surender Kumar Saini)

(D. Pharmacy, B.SC., M.SC. Preksha Meditation & Yoga, 3000hrs Intensive YTT at ICYER, India, MS Psychotherapy & Counselling)

Surender Saini, now known as Yogachariya Jnandev, was born into a typical Hindu family. He grew up under the guidance and blessings of his virtuous parents, loving and caring two brothers and a sister. This gave Jnandev a strong foundation for a yogic, ethical and moral lifestyle. He has also been greatly influenced by his late Nana (grandfather), who was a great bhajan singer and spiritual storyteller. He encouraged Jnandev to read the Ramayama, Mahabharata and other Hindu epic stories. This planted the seeds of spirituality, Hinduism and yoga in Jnandev's young mind.

Jnandev began his career as a Pharmacist, but he did not enjoy that for long. He found it to be not of much use in helping people to be healthy or happy. So he went back to further education. Jnandev had a great interest in science and hence went on to do his graduate in Maths, Physics and Chemistry. These studies have given Jnandev a much greater understanding of many yogic ideas and principals from a scientific perspective.

In 1995, during the Pharmacy course, Jnandev met with a friend who gave him initiation into some concentration practices, relaxation techniques and a few asanas or postures to learn hypnosis. After a few months of Trataka, relaxation practices and some visualisation, Jnandev felt drawn to learn more and more about Hatha Yoga, meditation and relaxation techniques and followed the teachings of various ashrams, yoga centres, yoga shalas as and when he could. Since then he tries to do his sadhana every day.

After graduation Jnandev decided to enter the civil service in India and was preparing for competition exams for it. During this period his sadhana also got deeper and deeper and he felt drawn to finding the true meaning of life through yoga. This quest brought Jnandev to Jain Vishwa Bharati University, Ladnun and in 2002 he completed MSC in Preksha Meditation and Yoga as a gold medallist. Here he was blessed by presence of his Guru, Sthita Prajna ji, who guided Jnandev on every level of his sadhana. During the course, Jnandev spent most of his time in one of the richest libraries, where he managed to read or study many original scriptures and manuscripts. This was the time when Jnandev also started to write. Since 2000, Jnandev has written many articles, and research papers in India. This was the beginning point of this yoga course.

Since then Jnandev has visited and lived in many ashrams and yoga institutes to learn, practice and grow in his sadhana. From 2003 till 2006 Jnandev worked in one of the most reputable schools in Jaipur (M.G.P.S, Vidyadhar Nagar, Jaipur). This gave Jnandev a new opportunity to explore various aspects of Hatha Yoga practices to benefit young children.

Jnandev learned, followed and taught various Hatha Yoga kriya sets, asanas and mudras from beginner to advanced levels during this time. Jnandev also completed a Masters in Psychotherapy and Counselling course (distance learning) in order to understand the mind from a modern perspective.

From 2006 to 2007, Jnandev, seeking to advance his own sadhana and yogic development, arrived at Ananda Ashram, Puducherry. The advanced yoga teacher training course under the guidance of his now Gurus, Ammaji Meenakshi Devi and Dr Ananda Balayogi Bhavanani, completed Jnandev's journey in search of true, authentic yoga. This intensive six-month course in Gitananda Rishiculture Ashtanga Yoga was a life-changing experience for Jnandev. His Guru, Ammaji, also gave the name and title 'Yogachariya Jnandev' to Surender at the end of course, which he uses in most parts of his life now.

All this time, Jnandev managed to not only do his sadhana regularly, but to keep writing about his understanding and experience of various practices, philosophical ideas and principles. After meeting his wife, Yogacharini Deepika, Jnandev moved to the UK in 2008. In 2009 he established Yoga Satsanga Ashram, Wales, UK and in 2010 started to run his first foundation course in Yoga compiled from all the writings and teachings Jnandev had been working on since 2000. Towards the end of this course Jnandev and Deepika decided to register the course as a Yoga Teacher Training course. This Yoga course primarily follows Gitananda Yoga, but also has a great input of teachings and blessings from Jain Vishwas Bharati, Hatha Yoga Guru Balendu Giriji, Mahavira Nathaji and many more divine souls. The blessings of Ammaji and Dr Ananda has kept Jnandev on this straight path of Yoga.

Yogachariya Jnandev met his wife Yogacharini Deepika at Ananda ashram. They have three lovely boys and growing up in the Ashram has helped them to grow and evolve every day. Since Jnandev came to UK Deepika has been a great guide and contributor to his yoga journey. Deepika has worked very sincerely in helping Jnandev to bring this course to present form. May the Divine and GURU (one who shows us path to self-realisation and guides us from darkness to light) bless us all on this path of yoga and help us to grow spiritually together. May the Divine and Guru give us the strength and courage to follow this path of discipline which can lead us to union of body-mind-soul. May the Divine bless us all with SAT-CHIT-ANANDA (divine love and bliss).

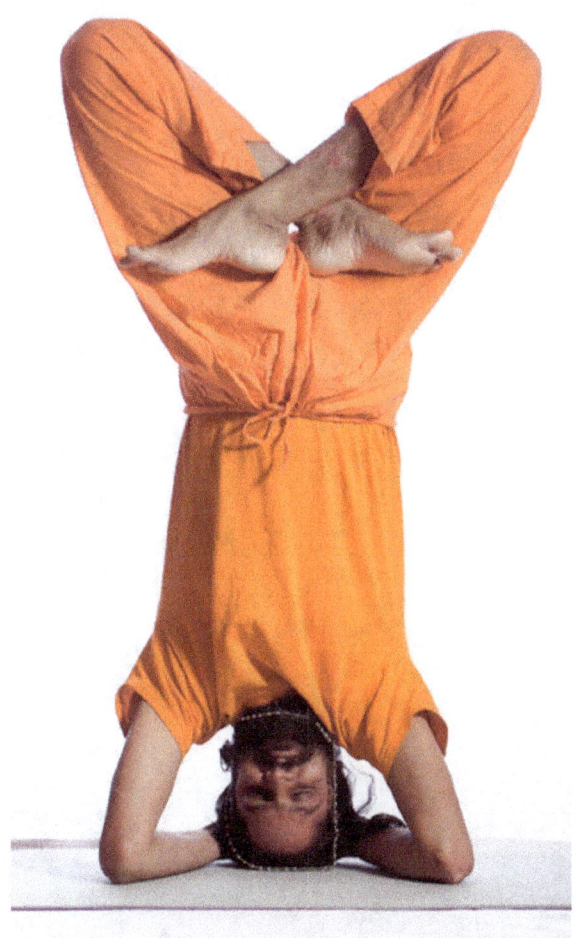

www.ingramcontent.com/pod-product-compliance
Lightning Source LLC
Chambersburg PA
CBHW071747080526
44588CB00013B/2178